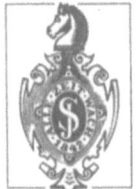

Springer-Verlag France S.A.R.L

ISCAMI 1

Integrated system for the Management
and Manipulation of Medical Images

Edited by J. Demongeot & A. Sousa Pereira

Springer-Verlag France S.A.R.L

Professeur J. Demongeot
Université Joseph-Fourier
Faculté de Médecine de Grenoble
Laboratoire d'informatique médicale
Domaine de la Merci
38700 La Tronche
France

Front picture: an ISCAMI processing itself.
    Frederic Berthommier TIMB Faculté de Médecine 38700 LA Tronche

---

© Springer-Verlag France 1991
Originally published by Springer-Verlag France, Paris, 1991

ISBN 978-2-287-59557-8   ISBN 978-2-8178-0883-3 (eBook)
DOI 10.1007/978-2-8178-0883-3

2918/3917/543210 — Printed on acid-free paper.

Foreword

The papers of the present book have been brought together after a COMAC-BME colloquium held in Aveiro (Portugal) in 1989 and supported by EEC. During this meeting, we have defined the concept of an Integrated System for Computer Assisted Management and Manipulation of Medical Images (ISCAMI), which does allow the multimodality matching of images coming from a PACS environment for diagnosis, therapy and medical education purposes. In order to achieve the building of such an ISCAMI workstation, we have concentrated our work in four sessions summarized as follows by their chairmen:

1) Prospective medical interest of PACS (Pr. Mattheus)

Several projects on PACS were presented, showing that the concept of PACS is moving gradually, but also that it is still not completely cheal how to organize the image department. Three levels of applications have been described concerning respectively the diagnosis, the therapy and the education, each of them having their technical, clinical, organizational and economical aspects. More specialized topics have been also presented: the study of the different factors having effect on image quality (detected by using a reference set of images), and a survey on the role of microscopic imaging which represents at this moment a different field of needs, not in clinical pressure.

2) Technical aspects of data manipulation in a PACS (Pr. Todd Pokropek)

A series of papers were presented about the method and problems of data compression. Particular concerns were those of the choice between reversible and non-reversible methods, and the choice of optimal method, adapted to the particular image to be encoded. In addition, the question of standards for other uses, such as HDTV and encoding « moving pictures » was presented, and the need for liaison with other standards groups stressed. Dr. Mattheus presented a survey of the PACS installation existing at AZ-VUB, and Pr. Lemke described the different types of networks that could be used for PACS, and the potential broadband ISD proposed for use in Berlin.

3) Generalized data bases and HIS-RIS-PACS interfaces (Pr. Lemke)

A survey and several specific aspects of image data base design were presented. The discussion emphasized the importance of distributed date base systems for PACS environments. PACS/RIS/HIS interface problems were presented by speakers from the Netherlands and FRG. Concepts for satisfactory solutions are avalaible. Some prototyping of PACS showing the advantage of an open system was demonstrated by a speaker from Sweden. A presentation on the aims of EUROPACS was followed by a discussion on general organizational support for PACS-like activities within and outside Europe.

4) Technical aspects of PACS and computer assisted use of images (Pr. Bakker)

In this session several papers were presented on developments that might add to the PACS concept value beyond improved archiving and communication of images. First image processing in the field of 3D and radiotherapy was considered. Some of the techniques were reported to be used already on a limited scale in clinical practice. The second half of the session dealt with possible use of robotics. First and overview was given of the developments in the UK as to robotics in the medical area. Next possibilities for computer assisted intervention were considered and the progress in this domain at Grenoble was reported. The session made it clear that the concerted action should not be restricted to mere archiving, communication and representation of images. Image processing deserves attention since basic PACS functions might bring such facilities in the realm of clinical application.

We hope that this beginning work will be concluded in a close future by the emergence of most of the functionalities devoted to an ISCAMI in its PACS environment. We thank very much Ms Geneviève Burnod for carefully preparing the final version of the book and Springer-Verlag France for publishing it.

A. Sousa Pereira
J. Demongeot

Table of Contents

Analysis of Radiologic Activity at Turku University Hospital in terms of Digital Data Transfer

Aaro Kiuru

Department of Radiology, Turku University Central Hospital
20520 Turku, Finland

The necessary time for the change from an analog radiologic imaging system to a PAC-system will be long in most hospitals. The turnover probably happens through the normal renewal of instrumentations over several years. The exceptions are only experimental and totally new X-ray departments. It is therefore clearly profitable to invest new X-ray instrumentation while keeping in mind their connection to existing and near future PAC-systems although many questions are still open.

Background

In Turku University Central Hospital (TUCH) an analysis of the present combined analog (thorax - bones - fluoroscopy etc) and digital (two CT, MR, DSA, lung imaging) imaging systems in terms of image volumes and data transfer rates has been made. The work covers both our four X-ray departments at the university hospital (UH) level and radiological activities at lower levels of the health care, namely in one local hospital (LH) and one health centre (HC). This report concerns the X-ray department A, where 73 % of all radiologic activity of TUCH was made in 1988.

The number of X-ray examinations in 1988 in the X-ray departments under study were the following:

HOSPITAL   no of examinations / 1988

- the UH level:

A-department	72 617
U-departement	38 003
Angio departement	2 593
Lung- departement(Paimio)	13 116
sum	126 329

- the LH level (Raisio):   14 018 (there are 5 others)
- the HC level (Naantali):   5 531 (there are 13 others)

Measurement and Results

We have at our disposal the statistics of X-ray examinations in 1988. They were classified according to the code of examinations and the X-ray laboratory. When the size of film-cassette (10 different cassettes were given the codes from 1 to 10) and the average number of films in each examination was known, it was possible to calculate the number of actually used films in each X-ray room as the function of film size. Therefore the total number of films (Fig. 1) and total film areas in each laboratory during 1988 was obtained.

When the assumption of 5 x 5 pixels per one mm2 on film and 12 bits of intensity (4096 gray shades, that is 2 bytes / pixel) in the AD-conversion is utilized, it is possible to reach the amount of image data transfer in GB between each local image archive and the departmental image archive. A plan of possible PACS-nodes and PACS-net at the radiology department A is shown in Fig. 2. This covers the activities in 1988 (with the total number of digital data, if all the films in Fig. 1 were digitized with the above mentioned pixel assumption) combined into six units, each including imaging devices in 1 or 2 X-ray rooms, one image work station (report) and one local digital archive. All units are connected to the image archive of this department (being probably simultaneously the digital image archive of the hospital) and via that further to other departments; surgery, polyclinics, bed wards.

It is worth while noticing that instead of the largest number of films used in skeletal work (62170 in Fig. 1), Fig. 2 shows that the largest storage capacity is needed in the thorax laboratory (330 GB).

From the distribution of patients entering to the X-ray department A during one week in 1987 (non published data) it can be found that about 30 % of the daily work is peaked between 8 and 9 a.m. Knowing also that 73 % of examinations in department A are performed between 7 and 15 daily, it is possible to obtain an estimate of peak transfer rates in Mbits/s. Figure 3. shows the individual maximum transfer rates and the total maximum transfer rate, about 1.2 Mbits/s. They occur thus between 8 and 9 a.m., when the new images are stored to the departmental (or hospital) image archive.

What about old images? They are needed by the X-ray technologist and the radiologist, when a new examination is carried out, interpreted and reported. A certain portion of patients in the hospital image archive has lot of images. But the average number of films is around 8 corresponding about 0.5 m2 of film (unpublished data) and therefore about 25 MB total digital storage with the pixel and byte assumptions given above. But what is important is that only the image or images of the former examination are normally needed during the present examination. This doubles the capacity space and transfer rates (old images are, however, often possible to prefetch during the earlier day or night), but very probably does not make it three times as large as shown in this investigation.

If instead of 0.2 x 0.2 mm2 pixel size one uses 0.1 x 0.1 mm2 pixel, all numbers concerning digital units above and in Fig. 2 and 3 must be multiplied with factor 4. The pixel size 0.1 x 0.1 mm2 is evidently necessary for thorax imaging, but 0.2 x 0.2 mm2 is sufficient for example for today's brain CT-images (150 mm / 512 is about 0.3 mm). Therefore the actual digital storage for new images is somewhere between the numbers given in this study and their four fold values.

The evident conclusion is that it is vital to know the parameters in present X-ray activity in order to plan, budget and invest with minor mistakes to digital picture archiving and communication systems.

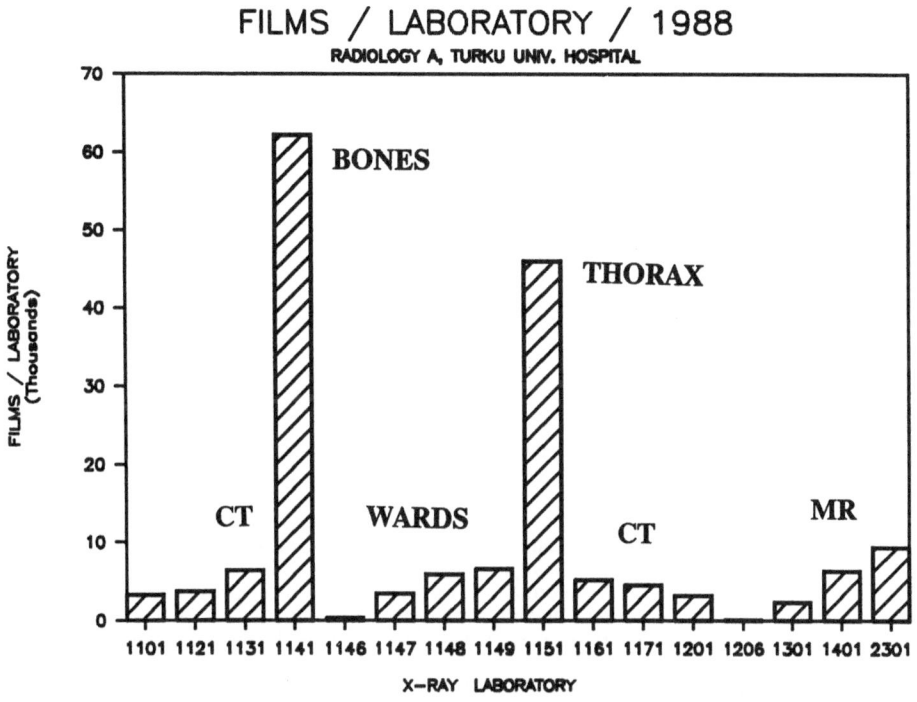

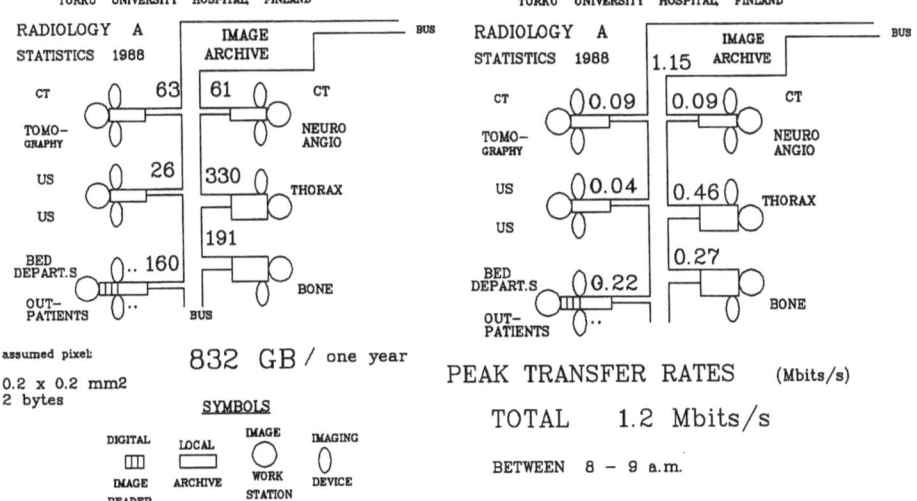

Clinical Radiology and PACS

Jean Claude KURDZIEL MD, Robert F. DONDELINGER MD
Dept. of Diagnostic and interventional Radiology
Centre Hospitalier - 4 rue Barblé
L- 1210 LUXEMBOURG

Introduction :

Since the early presentation of a digital network and storage system named Picture Archiving and Communication System (PACS) (1), substantial progress has been achieved in PACS technology and various components have appeared on the market. Small scale PACS, commercially available or custom made, have also been tested by many institutions worldwide.

Potential Archiving and communication improvements gained through a PACS, have raised a lot of enthousiasm among both the technological and medical communities.

Despite PACS is considered a promising step for adequate management of an increasing number of digital images, no hospital actually runs a complete functioning PACS network in the world. However, implementation of totally integrated systems will probably be attempted within the next few years.

There are many reasons why such a process has not yet been achieved :
- only a limited number of images are acquired in digital format in the actual daily work of any department of radiology
- the hard copy on film and the film itself has a strong historical position in the radiology department
- all the tasks that should be achieved by a digital management system in the radiology department, including those actually assumed by the film (acquisition, display, consultation, communication, education, research) are not precisely defined.

Image acquisition and image management (display, storage, communication) must be transferred from the actual film-based work to the future digital-based work, taking in account clinical needs, in order to raise PACS to a level of acceptable clinical and technical performance with reasonable costs. If general acceptance of the system can be gained, implementation will be possible in hospitals.

The image life - cycle

The medical images, basically produced in the radiology and nuclear medicine departments (which are joint in a medical imaging department in some hospitals) have a typical life-cycle from birth (image acquisition) to death (image destruction). The length of the image life-cycle depends on various factors (general hospital, teaching and research in university hopital, ...) among which legal obligations for film archiving duration is the most constraining and varies between countries.

Image acquisition

At present time about 25 % to 30 % of images are acquired in a digital format (MRI, CT,DSA, US, NM, DR). 70 % to 75 % of images are acquired on film . Even digitally acquired images are reproduced on film which supports their life-cycle.

In the radiology department, the film deserves all functions mentionned above except acquisition for digital modalities. The film is a practical compromise between the conflicting requirements of all those tasks. It may be replaced if all tasks are superseded at clinically acceptable levels, being economic and practical.

Many attempts have been made to digitize the conventional radiographic images acquired on film, among which fluoroscopic image digitization and storage phosphore screen systems are the most relevant. Both techniques show the following advantages: they fulfill the requirements of appropriate contrast (necessary for viewing) and greatest possible latitude (necessary for image acquisition). In that respect, they surpass the radiographic film. Spatial resolution of the film is adequate for diagnostic radiology and remains superior to that of digital radiography.

If image acquisition on films should be replaced by digital acquisition, the resulting images should contain all of the clinically relevant information. It is not established today that the higher contrast resolution and display potentials will compensate for the loss of spatial resolution of digital images compared with film images in all fields of application.

Many studies have been performed to determinate the appropriate pixel size for a digital radiographic image of the chest. A pixel size ranging from 0,33 mm (2) to 0.1 mm or even smaller (3) has been considered accurate. No standardized criteria were used for those studies. Varying acquisition parameters and different modalities for digitization (digital acquisition, digitization of film, reviews on screens and /or films) were used. Receiver operating characteristics (ROC) and modified ROC studies are presented with differences in study design. Furthermore, even if a non significant statistical difference exists between conventional and digital images in terms of performance in reading, medico-legal conflicts could be generated by false negative diagnoses, even if their number is minimal.

Image display

The film is the standard for image display in all radiology departments. Soft display is mostly used to monitor the digital examinations (MRI, CT, US...) and has not replaced hard-copy on film for routine diagnosis from digital modalities.

Soft display of images requires adaptation of the radiologists and clinicians, necessary for a broad base acceptance. Soft display should deserve the same functionality than films. It is crucial that all images of one particular examination (MRI, CT, DSA,...) could be visualized with full spatial resolution at time of reporting. Reviewing one image after the other might be time consuming and reading images with loss of spatial resolution might result in a loss of diagnostic accuracy.

It is also important that soft display will be used by the clinicians, who review the images which are processed in the radiology or nuclear medicine departments, because if hard copies are generated for communication of results and display for the clinicians, no reasonable economic advantage can be expected to justify PACS installation.

For soft display used by referring physicians, all the relevant clinical information should be present in the image. It is not established that non radiologist reviewers will accept a loss in image quality from lower quality workstations.

Soft display of medical images may be more problematic on the ward, except if mobile workstations could be developped at reasonable costs.

Image management

Processing

Wether the processing of digital images (windowing, filtering, edge enhancement...) will increase diagnostic accuracy by improving the perception of clinically important information has not been demonstrated for digital radiography until today. There are only few types of examinations in which the most powerful interactive image manipulations are medically justified (i.e. 3D examinations of the face for plastic surgery planning).

Many justifications have been proposed for image processing of standard radiographic examinations; the potential for reduction of radiographic exposures and increase of diagnostic yield are the most prominent. It is not yet demonstrated that interactive image processing reduces significantly the fraction of missed positive findings in diagnostic radiography. Even if this could be proved, the method should be less time consuming and more economic than double film reading by two radiologists or discussion with clinicians.

Processing is commonly used for CT or MRI images, including window selection, and measurements of size, distance, density or intensity. Image processing is also commonly used in

DSA for selection of the most significant subtracted images.

Image compression :

Image compression has been suggested to reduce the already large amount of digital data produced by a radiology department, and cope with their significant increase when total digital radiology will be introduced in daily practice.

Preliminary studies have estimated a production of 50 GB a day for a 540 bed hospital (4), with full data storage.

Image compression could reduce the archiving volumes and communication times on the image network.

Wether compression of medical images is acceptable from a clinical point of view is an unsolved question. Extensive research has to be driven in that area for all types of medical images using standardized image sets and ROC analyses

Image compression can be foreseen at various levels. Although selection of clinically relevant images by the radiologists is a common procedure for DSA and NM examinations, such a process is not routinely used for other digital or analogical modalities. However, image selection might represent the most significant way to reduce the amount of images to be manipulated later on. This process is called "*clinical compression*". Additional data decrease can be gained from "*localized compression*", which is a process of cancellation or significant irreversible compression of non clinically relevant information contained in one image. Further "*digital data compression*" can be performed on the reversible or irreversible modes. Evaluation of those modalities and especially their impact on diagnostic accuracy is mandatory, prior to their acceptance and introduction in clinical pratice. Initial false negative diagnoses are often recognized during review and initial data manipulation should never delete clinically important features.

Full data manipulation of medical images would be optimal, as no information is lost.

Considering the progress made in hardware, software and networks in the past decades one can assume that manipulation of full image data may become a reality on a routine basis in the future.

In the meantime, image compression to some degree, inspiring medical confidence, may partially solve the problem of processing such large amounts of data.

Reporting :

The radiologist analysizes a set of images and produces a report describing the radiologic findings and, in correlation with the clinical/biological status of the patient, gives a diagnostic impression of the patient's state of health or even concludes to the definite diagnosis. Clinical information on the patients are available when performing and/or reporting on one examination.

Film analysis on light boxes is common in any radiology department, as most radiologists presently prefer working with hard copies, even for digital acquisition modalities.

It is usual that previous films are reviewed for comparison with actual images. Correlation between different diagnostic imaging modalities are also performed at time of reporting on one particular examination (i.e CT and US). Therefore, images archived in a digital format should be fully restored for comparison (even a previous true negative image).

When radiologists will move from reporting on hard copies to soft display, the tools that will do that display should be interactive, easy to manipulate and meet the medical requirements previously stated, which means :
- to allow visualization of full resolution digital images, including digital radiography
- to allow visualization of all images of one examination with full information
- to guarantee the availability of relevant clinical and biological information.

Some examinations are reported on the site of image production (i.e., CT, MRI, ...).However, the possibility should be given to review images from all types of examinations on one workstation. The number of those reporting or review workstations has to be defined, according to the architectural and funtional organization of the radiology department.

Reporting from a workstation should also improve the report itself. Short vocal comments, cursor demonstrations could be registered together with the images and circulate with them.

Communication :

At present time, the film image is used for communication of information inside and outside the radiology department. The radiologic consultation includes both the images and the report. The referring physician gets the report and the images which contain the same information than those used by the radiologist for reporting. Communication is not limited today to a one-way transmission of images and reports. Interactive discussions between clinicians and radiologists on images or examinations are common in the radiology or clinical department.

Digital communication of images and reports is generally presented as a way of reducing delay between image acquisition and final use of the information by the referring physician. When networks will be installed in the hospital for communication of images and reports, clinicians will accept to use soft display in their office, providing response time of the PACS is acceptable and all clinical important information are available on the transmitted image.

PACS should permit interactive discussion i.e by telecommunication between the radiologist and the clinician, each being on his own workstation, both viewing the same images.

Archiving :

Archiving of medical images is an obligation. The requirements for archiving vary according to national legal and local hospital imperatives, according to the type of institution.

Legal requirements for archiving radiological images concern long term archiving and vary between european countries from 10 years to "eternal".

Even if general rules that apply to all institutions for archiving of medical images cannot be defined, several needs for image availability can be identified in clinical radiology. They can be defined as immediate, medium term and long term availability requirements.

In the image life cycle, immediate availability can be defined as the period between image acquisition and clinical exploitation. It comprises analysis of the images by the radiologist, reporting, and communication to the refering physican. During this process, the film image is immediately available to the radiologist and secondary transmitted to the clinician with the radiological report within 1 hour to 2 days, depending on the institution, type of patient (outpatient - in hospital) and type of examination, the process being shorter for examinations which do not need an extensive review of images,. No archiving is actually performed during that period with the film image, which is handled and serves as archival medium.

Digitization of the process during immediate availability needs performant archiving media, with short or nil response times on an efficient network . If this cannot be achieved, hard copies of images will undoubtfully be produced at high rates and serve for display, communication and consultation.

It is determinant during this initial phase that all the clinical relevant information be kept present in the image

Medium term availability can be understood as the period between initial clinical exploitation of the images and final archiving after full exploitation. During that period, the images are used either for comparison with previous examinations of the same type or for correlation with other examinations (i.e., US and CT). Availability of images in the radiology department must be guaranteed with response times less than 15 seconds and full clinical significance.

For inpatients, the requirements are the same than for the immediate availability time period. For outpatient, it seems difficult to by-pass the hard-copying process for image communication.

Long term availability is defined as the period after the active medical history has been solved or when treatment of the outpatient is achieved or when the inpatient has left the hospital. According to the use that will be made of the images in the future, various concepts can be stressed :

1. Pressure for availability of the images for follow-up or in case of recurrent disease is unpredictable and therefore no loss of relevant clinical information in the images could be accepted.

2. When a true negative image is reviewed to evaluate the moment of appearance and speed of development of a pathological process, any loss in the initial image at storage and restitution might be unsignificant. However if the initial image led to a false negative report, this might only be discovered at reviewing and therefore, full restoration of information from the initial image is determinant.

3. Whatever the information contained in the image is , it may be used later on for research and/or educational purposes. No compromise in reduction of the initial information is then acceptable.

Considering response delays, they should be nil or kept within seconds for immediate availability, within 10 - 15 seconds for medium term availability and below 1 minute for long term availability ; previous selection of cases and storage in an active file allowing fast work makes this possible.

Conclusions :

When digital radiography will reach confidence levels of technical and medical maturity and will be installed in the radiology department, the need for PACS will become stronger and attempts will be made to implement total systems. Those systems won't however be limited to the initial description of PACS, they must perform image management (archiving, communication) and manipulation (processing, compression, assisted reporting with cursor, vocal comments,...) and also be able to communicate with HIS and RIS or better, be integrated in those systems.

Ergonomics of the daily work in the radiology department must be clearly identified to be transferred in the digital mode. Precise medical requirements and expectations have to be defined by expert radiologists, regarding the ergonomics of clinical radiology. Scientific evaluation of digital radiography such as the persistent clinically important information in the images at acquisition, during processing and communication, and after compression is another determinant task to gain acceptability.

Finally, PACS allowing also image management and manipulation will be implemented in the radiology departments, providing they are able to replace display, communication, consultation, archiving, educational and research capacities of the film, in a more efficient and economic way, improving patient care.

References

1). 1st International Conference and Workshop on Picture Archiving and Communication System (PACS) for Medical Applications- Newport Beach *Proc. SPIE*. 1982;138

2). Lams P.M., Cocklin M.L: "Spatial resolution requirements for digital chest radiographs : a ROC study of observer performance in selected cases".*Radiology*. 1986;158 , pp 11 -19

3). MC Mahon H., Vyborny C.J., Metz C.E., Doi K, Sadetti V., Solomon S.L.: "Digital radiography of subtle pulmonary abnormalities : a ROC study of the effect of pixel size on observer performance". *Radiology*. 1986;158, pp 21-26

4). Templeton A.W., Cox G. G., Dwyer S.J.III: "Digital image management networks : current status".*Radiology* . 1988; 169, pp 193 - 199

Advantages of picture archives and communication system (PACS) in health care in great oporto. A multihospital project.

J.A Veiga-pires and J. Almeida-pinto
departments of imagiology, gaia medical centre (Santos Silva hospital) and Santo Antonio hospital, Oporto. Portugal

Introduction

This paper presuposes an informed knowlege of the picture archives and communication system (PACS) which, therefore, shall be only discussed in its functional and not structural aspects.

PACS in its original concept is an imminently imagiology weighted system, because already 30% to 40% of all the imagies generated in a general up-to-date department are digital. Howerer, PACS obvious potentialities in the matrix interplay of the whole socio-economical fenomena, opens up a wide field of development and research. As a system at the cutting edge of technology PACS is a tool of the future desirable as from today.

The digital fabric core of modern imagiology propiciated the genesis and development of PACS as a promising and certainly revolutionary path to the knowledge of the world and social evolution.

Thus the propose of this paper is to discuss the impact of PACS in imagiology, therapeutic and interventional Radiology, Nuclear Radiology and Radiationtherapy-Oncology planning and interaction in terms of patient management and health care policy and economics.

By the integrating key hospitals of the great Oporto health care region through PACS networks a twofold benefit can be derived, in the social and in the economical realms.

Portugal is beaconning out of the twighlitght that bridges the developing and the developed countries communications' wise which makes her an excellent test best for the evaluation of the impact of PACS. Great Oporto is an agraved picture of the whole country because of its current populational and services growth upsurge with dynamics altogether suigeneris because they run counter severe communication bottle necks, be them roads or telephon networks.

Great oporto and her central hospitals

Great Oporto and her area of influence comprises about 40% of Portugal's 10m inhabitants. Most of this population concentrate in an area of about 50 milles radius, strangulated by all kinds of communication bottle necks whereby the commercial cruising speed can be as low as fives milles per hour. The differentiated health care facilities are attended to by four central hospitals and a well hardware equiped cancer hospital seconded by regional hospitals of varying degrees of care sofistication, most of them with teaching responsabilities, either pre-and/or post-graduate. The central and regional hospitals are on the whole serviced by underdimensioned imaging departments lacking in state-of-art technology and staff and relying on obsolete hardly reliable patient records systems. The clinical, technical, scientific and managerial intercourse among these hospitals is negligeable.

Howerer, within this framework there are relatively highly effective imaging departments wich are the driving force behind a surge of renovation that must come with Portugal's integration in the EEC.

PACS and health care in great oporto

As means of integration of departments of imagiology, PACS and its informatic networks come as the tool that will make possible to overcome the current inefficacy predicament caused by structural shortcomings and the above mentioned communication bottle necks the health care system suffers of, compouded by lack of adequated financing. Investment in PACS is stil today rather high ($100,000) seen in terms of its implementation in a single institution, even if a central teaching hospital, which may see its development budget overcome by the initial costs. However, integrated in a network the costs would be significantly reduced on quantity buying thus minimized by the sharing among several institutions.

The great Oporto PACS Project here advocated is intended to loop in the following institutions: Departments of Imagiology of Santos Silva hospital (Gaia medical centre), Santo antonio hospital (Oporto), Vale do Sousa Medical Centre, Portuguese Institute of Oncology (Oporto), S. Marcos Hospial (Braga) and Hæmodynamics Laboratory (S. Joao Hospital, Oporto) to start with.

Community of filing systems, speed of and high density knowledge transfer, maximization of haevy hardware utilization, higher degree of work discipline and responsability towards the patient will induce the passage of the existing hospitals from an amorphous self- and territory centrered institutions into a much more efficacious healthcare network with significante socio-economical benefits. Moreover, the knowledge transfer function would have a prime elective influence on the teaching that goes on dayly in these institutions.

Report on Digital Video Transmission Activities at INESC-NORTE

Antonio T. Gaspar, Manuela S. Pereira, M. Teresa Andrade, Nuno Vasconcelos,
A. Pimenta Alves

1. Introduction

Activity in the area of Digital Video Transmission started in 1986. Until now this effort has been carried essentially as part of the SIFO Project.
This report describes past and present work and discusses some of the future perspectives.

2. Completed Developments

2.1 Parallel Video Codec

The activity started with the development of a Parallel Video Codec. Two evaluation boards were designed and built, around TRW's TDC1048 and TDC1016, and performed the analog-to-digital and the digital-to-analog conversions. These boards were connected back-to-back producing a Digital Video Codec with parallel transmission.

For the low-pass filter various topologies and types were tested and the filter chosen was a two-stage third-order Chebychev active filter with a cutoff frequency of 6.8 MHz.

Tests performed in January 1987 showed that the amplitude of the video signal was within ± 5% of the normalized value and all phases of the crominance were within ± 3%.

These boards were used to digitize composite video signals (PAL) at up to 8 bit/sample and up to 20×10^6 samples/second, in order to evaluate subjective effects on image quality.

2.2 153.6 Mbit/s Composite Video Codec

This Codec was developed as a means to test other SIFO subsystems, at a stage when the MUX/DEMUX generating the 153.6 Mbit/s frame were not ready. It uses the previously mentioned evaluation boards to accomplish the A/D and D/A conversions.

The composite video signal (PAL) is sampled at a sampling rate of 13.568 MHz with 8 bit/sample and coded in linear PCM. The digital video data is multiplexed with a digital audio channel (2048 Kbit/s), with the 153.6 Mbit/s frame synchronization word, with 139.264 Mbit/s frame synchronization word and with the empty slot signal. It is important to note that the digital video data and the associated digital audio data are formatted as a 139.264 Mbit/s frame inside the 153.6 Mbit/s frame. A fast FIFO working as an elastic buffer is used to accommodate the difference between the video data production rate (13.568 MHz) and the multiplexing rate (19.2 MHz). A sequential controller determines the timing for the insertion of the different signals. The last operation is the parallel-to-serial conversion made with a 10KH ECL device.

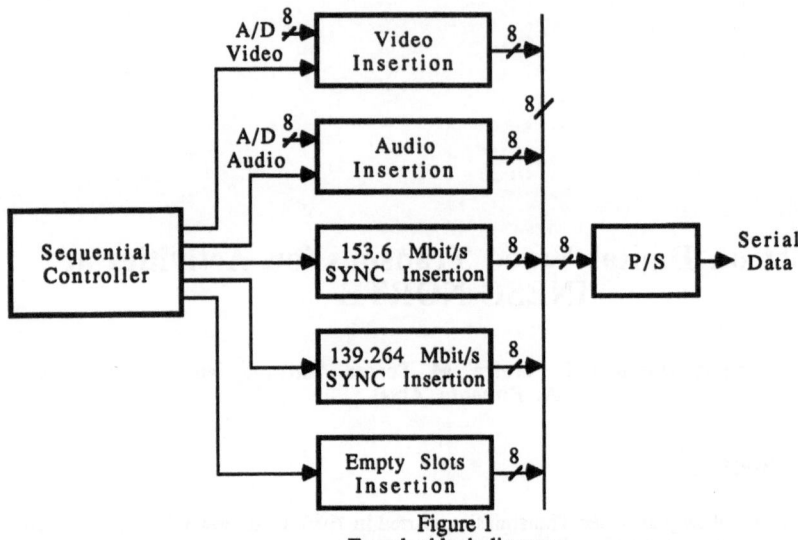

Figure 1
Encoder block diagram.

In the decoder the complementary operations are performed. A sequential controller is also used in this unit.

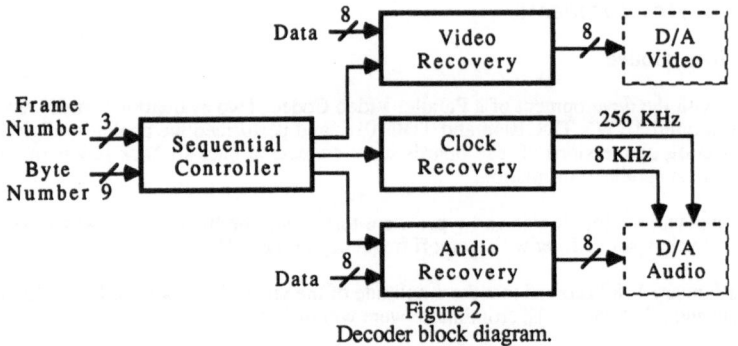

Figure 2
Decoder block diagram.

This development was completed and tested with success in June 1988, and it was demonstrated during the Preliminary Demonstration of the SIFO Project, during July 1988.

The quality obtained was very good. The main limitation of this Codec comes from the fact that it requires synchronization between the sampling clock, that must be locked to the colour carrier frequency, and the network clock.

2.3 139.264 Mbit/s Components Video Codec

This Codec was designed for the distribution of digital video in the SIFO network. It allows the transmission of a three-component video signal and the associated stereo audio channel at a 139.264 Mbit/s rate.

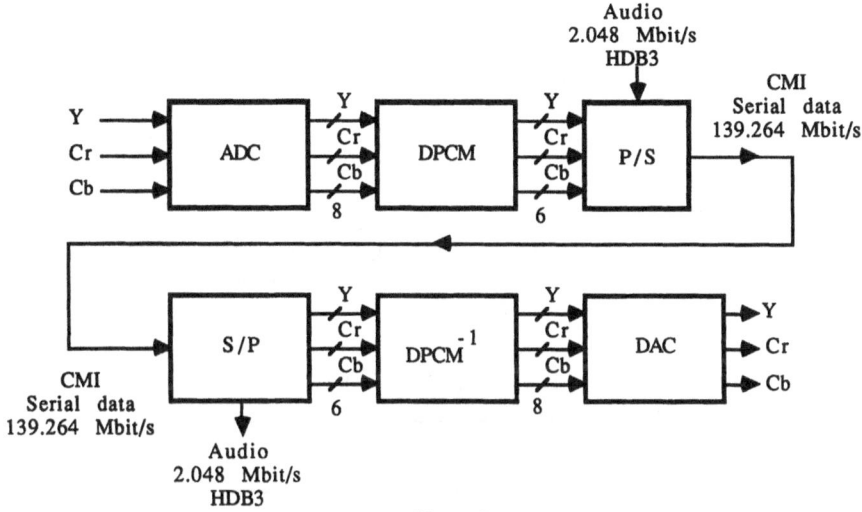

Figure 3
139.264 Mbit/s Codec block diagram.

The ADC and DAC interfaces follow the CCIR's Rec. 601. The luminance signal (Y) is sampled at a 13.5 MHz rate and the colour difference signals (Cr, Cb) are sampled at 6.75 MHz rate (Level 4:2:2).

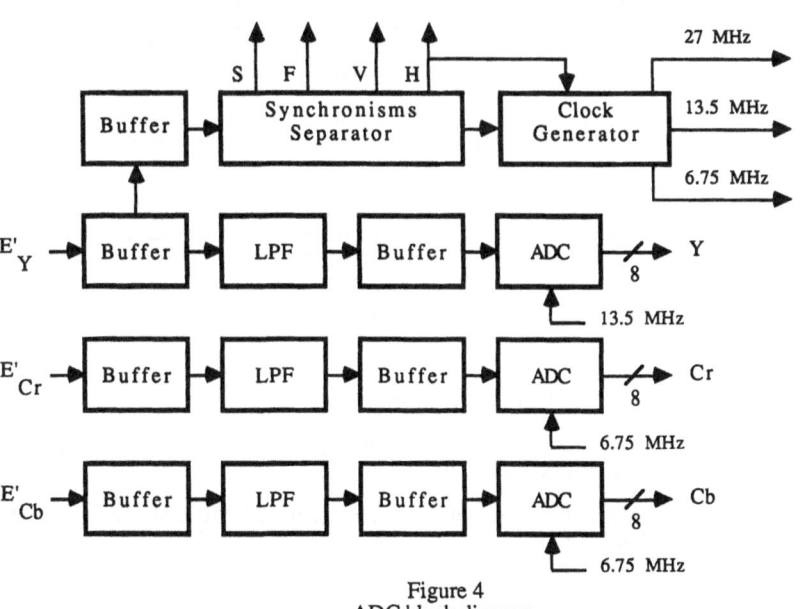

Figure 4
ADC block diagram.

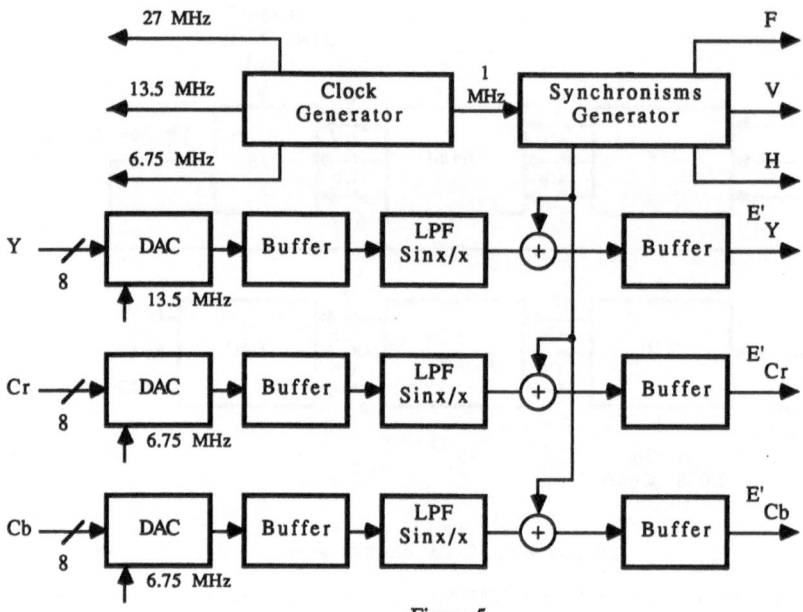

Figure 5
DAC block diagram.

The bit rate obtained is 216 Mbit/s and it must compressed in order to obtain the desired transmission rate (139.264 Mbit/s). This is accomplished using the hybrid DPCM coding method proposed by Van Bull, converting 8-bit PCM words into 6-bit DPCM words and eliminating the video signal horizontal blanking period. The prediction is made using the previous sample.

As the data rate produced is different from the transmission rate, it is necessary to accommodate the difference between them. This is accomplished with a stuffing scheme implemented with elastic buffers.

The audio is received in a 2.048 Mbit/s frame and is formatted with the video data for transmission. The frame used is a 139.264 Mbit/s similar to one of the frames recommended for multiplexing purposes in the Rec. G.700 series. CMI code is used for transmission.

This development is now completed and tests have already started at the subsystem level.

2.4   2 Mbit/s Video Codec

This Codec was designed to provide transmission of monochrome video pictures over 2048 Kbit/s digital channels, with a picture quality sufficient for surveillance purposes. It accepts one standard monochrome or colour (PAL) video signal with 625 lines and 50 field/s. Processing is reduced in order to keep the costs reduced and development time short.

The signal is bandlimited to 2 MHz and sampled at a frequency of 5 MHz, locked to the video waveform, producing 320 samples per complete line. Only 256 samples per active line are transmitted. The signal is coded with uniformly quantized PCM with 6 bit per sample.

In order to transmit this video signal in a 2048 Kbit/s channel the signal must be further compressed. To achieve this the video blanking periods are not transmitted (but the information of their temporal location is kept for future insertion of timing reference codes) and the digitized video signal is vertically and temporally subsampled and coded in DPCM with 3 bit per sample. As a result, only 286 lines per frame (or 143 lines per field) and only 8 frames per second (or 16 fields per second) are transmitted.

After these operations the video data is applied to a buffer memory whose function is to smooth the irregular data rate and adapt it to the constant bit rate of the 2.048 Mbit/s stream. In this buffer memory the video data is expanded along the time of the suppressed lines, frames and video blanking signals.

Timing reference codes must be inserted at this point to insure the proper recovery at the receiving end of the video signal format. They consist of a sequence of three 6-bit words, being the two first ones a fixed identification preamble with PCM forbidden values and the third one containing information about video synchronization and odd/even field identification.

The data stream is then formatted in a frame according to the CCITT G.700 Recommendations.

This Codec is now fully completed and tested.

This Codec will be used for the study of image transmission in a packet network environment.

3.   Future work

Work is now aiming at three main objectives, shortly described below.

3.1   34 Mbit/s Video Codec

Once the 140 Mbit/s Codec tests are concluded, work will start on a 34 Mbit/s Video Codec, with quality adequate for video distribution. The processing will follow ITU available Recommendations. For the processing particular attention will be given to the FDCT (Fast Discrete Cosine Transform).

3.2   Variable bit rate

There is a growing interest in variable bit rate codecs, to be used in ATM networks (Asynchronous Transfer Mode). The development of a VBR Codec in cooperation with other INESC groups involved in network aspects, is now under preparation.

3.3   px64kbit/s Codecs

This type of codec will shortly be used for image transmission in a number of experimental projects. Participation in a special program, supported by the Telecom Operators, is now being prepared, aiming at the development of such a Codec, with a flexible architecture.

Experiments will continue with the 2 Mbit/s Surveillance Codec developed.

Principles for PACS Evaluation

Dr. Eng. Paolo GIRIBONA
Centre for the Evalution of Biomedical Equipemt-Ce. V.A.B
Research Area of Trieste - Padriciano, 99 - 34100 TRIESTE- ITALY
Tel. + 39. 40. 226662 - Fax + 39. 40. 226698

1   PACS Technology

"Picture archiving & communication system" (PACS) refers to the method of managing a vast amount of radiological images and information by use of the capabilities of a computer network consisting of many subsystems for the purpose of archiving, distributing, communicating, displaying and processing the image data throughout the Radiology services and hospital complex.

The integration of digital imaging systems and advanced computer technologies has opened new possibilities in managing diagnostic images with a consequent improving of diagnostic accuracy, reduction of x-ray dose to patients, optimization of diagnostic process, reduction of costs, and improvement of organization.

The major functions of a PACS are to capture images from the acquisition devices (radiological equipment, digital imaging equipment, etc.), to transmit and store images, to provide the means to display and manipulate images, and to provide image archival capability.

In examining the requirements for a PACS and discussing possible architectures for such a system, a number of logical subsystems can be identified.

While the actual subsystem boundaries may not be so clearly defined, the subsystems that it is possible to identify at present are :

- capture points, where images and text initially enter the system
- user workstations, where images and cases are viewed and reports generated
  through the Radiology Information System
- communication network, consisting of image data and text data transmission
  facilities
- data and images storage, organized hierarchically
- a structured data base containing both images and text data connected to the R.I.S.and / or to
  the Hospital Information System

2   Assessment of PACS.

For PAC systems to be clinically accepted, they must prove their technical, clinical and economic merit.

Technical issues to be confronted can be grouped into six categories: image quality, image archiving, imaging systems and interfaces, communication networks, workstations, radiology information systems.

Main clinical and economic issues to be archieved should be :

- savings in films
- savings in consumables associated with films

- reduction in lost and misplaced films and reports
- reduction of exposures because of the ability to process images
- improved diagnostic accuracy because of image procesingf and ability to associate other clinical data with image data
- faster diagnosis, with possible shorter length of stay
- increased efficiency of departmental operations
- savings in capital costs for darkrooms and storage space
- saving in archiving personnel

From a general point of view, the introduction of PACS should allow a great improvement of organization of Radiology Departments and Hospitals, communication with remote areas and extension of diagnostic facilities.

PACS technology is still developing. At present, such systems are quite expensive and it is difficult to evaluate their benefits. As they mature technologically, benefits will become clearer and will be possible to do careful assessments.

However, it seems clear that PACS represent the future of radiology and medical imaging, and their introduction in the hospital environment in the next few years will be unavoidable.

A reasonable strategy for a national policy in this field is to encourage the assessment of PACS technology through the experimentation of prototype systems in several reference Hospitals, collecting data concerning clinical, technical and economic aspects .

2.1   Technological Evaluation

The aspects to be considered for a technical asessment of PACS are related both to performance criteria and to requirements for integration in the existing situation (imaging devices, health information systems, public telecommunication networks, etc.).

Main issues should be the following :

- Technical perfomances of the system :
Image quality, speed, workstation capabilities, archiving media, network performances, etc.

- Integration of the system with existing imaging devices :
TV frame grabbers, digital interfaces availability (non-standard, ACR-NEMA, etc.)

- Integration of the system with RIS and HIS :
interfaces, data format, access to operating system, etc.

- Compatibility with European communication standards : V35 - 48 kb/s, T2 - 2.048 Mb/s, etc.

2.2   Clinical Evaluation :

The evaluation of PACS from a clinical point of view involves a direct comparison with conventional diagnostic activity carried out on films.

However, not only image quality parameters should be taken into account but also changes on diagnostic efficiency related to PACS capabilities (direct access to images, transmission of images, processing, etc.).

Main issues to consider should be:

- Clinical acceptability of the system
- Ease of use (user interfaces)
- Diagnostic efficacy (CRT vs. film)

- Diagnostic efficiency

2.3   Organizational Evaluation :

The assessment of impact of a PAC System on the organization of a Radiology System is a crucial issue for other evaluations (economic, clinical, etc.).

The main aim of such evaluation should be to perform an analysis of how organization and management of operations in a Radiology Dept. are affected by the intoduction of PACS.

Fundamental phases of the evaluation can be the following :

- to build a general and comprehensive model of the Radiology System
- to identify the functions, activities and flows that can be affected by PACS
- to evaluate quantitatively the impact of PACS on each of such entities.

2.4   Economic Evaluation

One of the evaluation to be conducted for a complete assessment of PACS in the health care system is the analysis of the financial impact of this technology from both a theoretical and an actual experience perspective.

The most of methods of economic analysis use finances as the unit of objective measurement. On the other hand, cost effectiveness analysis is generally less objective but takes into consideration other significant affectiveness considerations in addition to cash flows.

Main issues to take into account should be :

- Costs of equipment
- Costs of personnel
- Costs of materials
- Costs of archiving
- System throughput
- System reliability

3. Experimentation of PACS in Italy : Trieste PACS Project

In order to assess the impact of PACS technology on health structures, a project of experimentation of a PAC system has been planned in 1987 at the Local Health Unit of Trieste (U.S.L. n.1 Triestina).

The U.S.L. n.1 is the administration of the four public hospitals of Trieste (2,500 beds, 4 Radiology Departments, about 250, 000 diagnostic imaging examinations/ year) delivering health care services to a population of about 260 000 inhabitants.

The long-term goal of the project is the realization of a metropolitan PACS network connecting the four hospitals and allowing the exchange of diagnostic images between them.

3.1 Present Configuration

A PAC System (CommView by AT &T and Philips) has been installed (September 1988) in the Radiology Dept. of Cattinara Hospital. The elements of the system are the following (fig.1) :

- DMS - Data Management System : central storage system (3.2 Gbyte on magnetic disks + 2Gbyte optical disk drive) and processor (Motorola 68020) for all images and patient data. The DMS communicates with the other devices of the system via a Network Communication Module which transmits images locally through fiber optics (40 Mb/s) and remotely through data transmission lines (T2 - 2.048 Mb/s or V35 - 48kb/s).

- AM- Acquisition Module : captures and digitizes the video signals from 5 digital scanning devices (MRI, CT, DSA and 2 Ultrasounds). Patient information is entered into the system via a

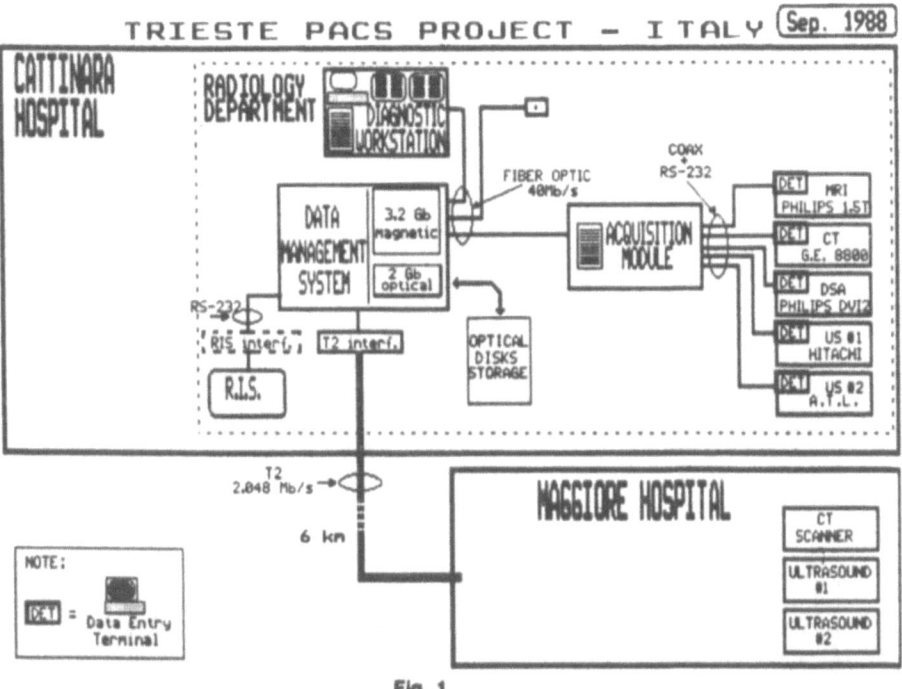

Fig. 1

Fig. 1

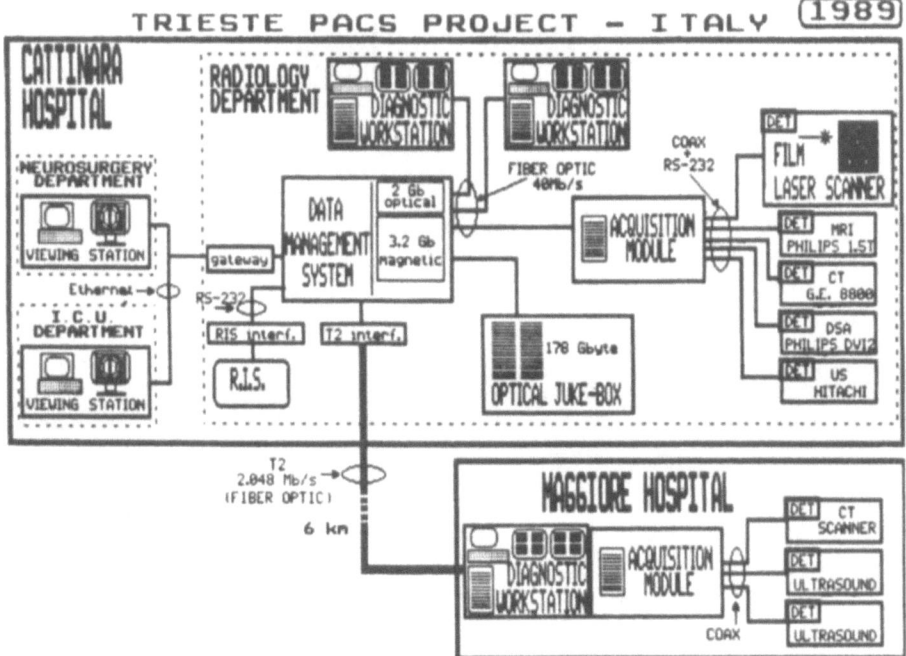

Fig. 2

TRIESTE PACS PROJECT – ITALY 199?

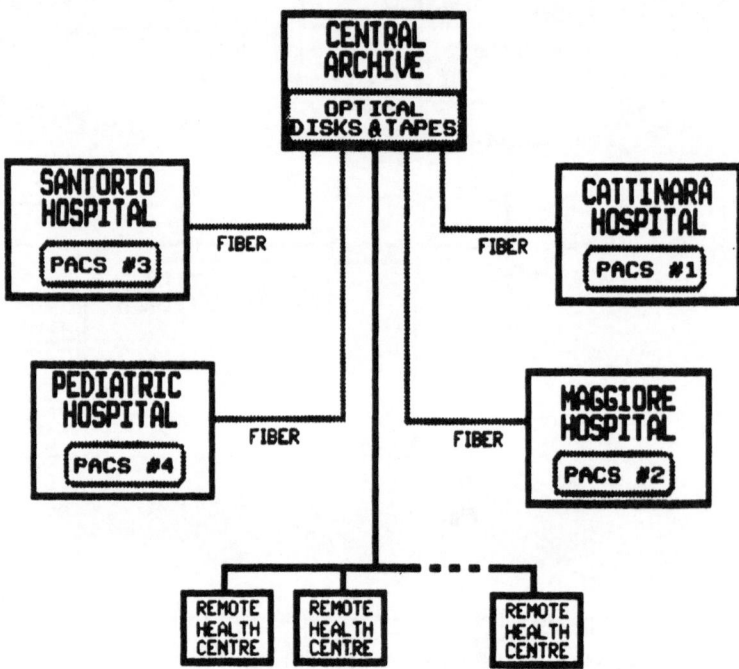

Fig. 3

Data Entry Terminal placed in each diagnostic room. Image matrix sizes are 512 x 512 x 8 bit.

- DW - Diagnostic Workstation : retrieves images and reports. Presently it is based on 2 1024 x 1024 hi-res screens with 4 images/screen.

Some basic manipulations of images are allowed (zoom, windowing, image move, etc).

A previously existing RIS (Radiology Information System) is going to be interfaced to the DMS trough a one-way RIS interface (from RIS to PACS). A communication line (T2 - 2.048 Mb/s) has been installed by the national telephone company (S.I.P.) between the Radiology Depts. of Cattinara Hospital and Maggiore Hospital (about 6 km).

3.2 Level of Utilization

The present configuration is widely used by the radiologists involved in digital diagnostic techniques (CT, MRI, DSA, Ultrasound).

All diagnostic activities on CT and DSA images are presently carried out on the PACS workstation. As far as ultrasounds are concerned, only the images of patients candidated for a subsequent CT, MRI or DSA examination are entered into the PACS and used for comparative multi-modality diagnosis. This is mainly due to the fact that, in Italy, ultrasound examinations are performed by physicians and diagnosis and reporting are performed at the moment of examination.

All images from MRI are entered into PACS ; however, the MRI scanner has been installed in January 1989, and presently it is in a preliminary stage of use (2-3 patients/day).

3.3 PACS Evaluation Activity

Some researches are currently under development in order to assess this new technology. The project involves a large number of people including radiologists, clinical engineers, data base experts, imaging physicists, health economy specialists.

The main goals of the assessment are :

Clinical Evaluation (Dept. of Radiology - University of Trieste)

- An experiment of comparison of diagnostic efficacy on CRT screen vs. conventional film has been carried out by four radiologists on about 100 Ct brain examinations (2 observations of the same clinical case with a time interval of 1 month) - Final results are going to be statistically analized.

- An experiment of contrast-detail perception is under development using computer generated patterns containing a random distribution of objects of different size and contrast with a variable amount of noise.

Technological Evaluation (Center for the Evaluation of Biomedical Equipment - Research Area of Trieste)

- A technical report, analyzing technical problems for the integration of a PACS in an existing Radiology Dept., is under development. Problems related to interfacing of PACS to existing aquipment, network installation, safety of data, hardware limitations, etc., are presently analyzed.

Requirements of communication with the external world will be defined on the basis of presently available resources (PACS-RIS communication, image transmission through public lines, access to archived images by external image- processing devices, etc.)

Organizational Evaluation (Dept. of Electronics and Informatics - University of Trieste)

- A research is in progress ofr the evaluation of impact of PACS on the organization of a Radiology System. The aim of this research is to analyze how organization and management of operations in a Radiology Dept. are affected by the introduction of PACS.

The method that is followed is based on 3 phases :

- building of a general model of the Radiology System

- identification of functions, actions and flows affected by PACS

- quantitative evaluation of PACS impact on each of such entities

Economic Evaluation (Ce. R. G. A. S. - "Bocconi" Economy University, Milan)

An agreement has been stipulated between the Hopital Administration of Trieste and Ce.R.G.A.S. of Milan for the Evaluation of economic impact of PACS (Ce.R.G.A.S. is a research and service division within "Bocconi" University dealing with economic studies on Public Health Institutions).

Cost analysis will be based on a previous study (carried out on a 3-year period : 1986-88) analyzing all cost components of Radiology Dept.s in the Hospitals of Trieste.

Main issues to be taken into account will be : costs of equipement, personel, materials and archiving ; dependence of such parameters on time required to perform actions ; analysis of trend of diagnostic imaging examinations (digital vs. conventional x- ray).

3.4 Short-Term Configuration

In a short while (june 1989, fig.2) the system will be further expanded by the acquisition of a high resolution Diagnostic Workstation (2 hi-res monitors- 20 images/screen in review mode), two Result Viewing Stations (to be installed in I.C.U. Dept . and Neurosurgery Dept.), one Diagnostic Workstation + Acquisition Module (to be installed in the Radiology Dept. of another Hospital 6 km away, connected to the main system through an optical line T2 -2.048 Mb/s), one film laser scanner and one optical juke-box (89 plates x 2Gbyte)

3.5 Long-Term Configuration

The final goal of the project is the implementation of a large area metropolitan PACS connecting the four main Public Hospitals of Trieste and some Remote Health Centers to a central archive (fig.3). This archive should collect images coming from the four Hospitals and allow a direct access to images from each Radiology Departement and from referring doctors in Remote Health Centers.

The project has some interesting aims :

- To improve the efficiency of the image archiving and retrieval process ;
- To interface PACS of different manufactures, pushing them to a standardization of communication interfaces ;
- To identify requirements for a large area network (using public telecommunication lines) suitable for exchange of medical images

.References

Mun S.K., Benson H. : "Fast-paced progress in computers ensures feasibility of PACS". *Diagnostic Imaging*.1987; nb 4, pp 106-116.

Greberman M., Gitlin J.N.: "Teleradiology / the relationship to PACS". *Proc. of Documed Europe 87* -Amsterdam-1987

Tiemann J.: "Picture archiving and communication systems (PACS) ": State of the art and future project *Proc. of Documed Europe 87*-Amsterdam-1987

Wendler T. : "Advanced image display in radiology." *Proc. of Documed Europe 87*-Amsterdam-1987

Williams A.R.: " A fibre optic communication network for teaching clinical medicine." *Proc. of Documed Europe 87*-Amsterdam-1987

Banata H.D., Behney C.J.: "Policy form*ulation and technology assessment*" .*Proc. of Documed Europe 87*- Amsterdam-1987

Van Beekum W.T., Banta H.D. : "policy implications of picture archiving and communication systems." *Proc. of Documed Europe 87*-Amsterdam-1987

Technical Specifications for a Hospital Based Digital Imaging Network. MITRE Corp., Mc Lean, VA, U.S.A., 1986

Digital Imaging Storage and Retrieval in the 1980s. *J. Health Care Technology*, 1984 ; 1, pp 13-38

Mun S.K., Elliot L.P., Benson H.R. : "Development and operational evaluation of PACS network at Georgetown University." *Progress Report*, Georgetown University, Washington D.C..1988

Oosterwijk H.J.: "Philips Medical Systems : PACS implementation : a tailored approach." Medical Imaging, *Proc. SPIE* 767. 1987; pp 752-757

Vanden J., Cyvinski J., Zerlag C.T. : "Cost analysis of present methods of image management." Medical Imaging, *Proc. SPIE* .1987; 767, pp 758-764

Bijl K., Koens M.L., Bakker A.R., de Valk J.P.J.: "Medical PACS and HIS : integration needed." Medical Imaging, *Proc. SPIE* .1987; 767, pp 765-770

O'Malley K.G., List J.S.: "Quality evaluation of images displayed on the AT&T "CommViev" system at Abbott Northwestern Hospital." Medical Imaging, *Proc. SPIE*. 1987; 767, pp 782-786

Wang Y. et al. : "Summary of compatibility of the ACR-NEMA imaging and communication standard." Medical Imaging, *Proc. SPIE*. 1987; 767, pp 819-822

Bakker A.R., Didden H., de Valk J.P.J., Bijl K. : "Traffic load on the image storage component in a PACS." Medical Imaging, *Proc. SPIE* .1987; 767, pp 824-830

Ivie M.E. : "Future trends and requirements for data bases in the PACS environment." Medical Imaging, *Proc. SPIE* .1987; 767, pp 839-843

Tobes M.C., Shonfeld S.M. : "Teleradiology operations within a PACS environment." Medical Imaging, *Proc. SPIE* .1987; 767, pp 849-852

Bravar D. et al.: " Costi ed attivita' di alcuni servizi di radiodiagnostica." Rapporti Finali AC. MA. GEST., Consiglio Nazionale delle Ricerche, Roma. 1987

Evaluation in PACS: Physical Tests and Clinical Test Data Sets.

A. Todd-Pokropek**, R. M. Dawood*
* St Mary's Hospital, London
** University College London

Introduction

There are two special problems in achieving a working PACS system, firstly capturing the data, and secondly displaying the resulting images. Unless these problems can be successfully resolved, all the rest of any PACS network is without practical clinical value, which is not to say that the problems associated with the management of such networks, the communications between the PACS components and the PAS, etc are without difficulties themselves. It was these input and output stages that we decided to address. Since data capture from CT scanners, MRI devices, and other digital systems is essentially an electronic and software problem, it was also decided to confine the area of study to conventional (film) radiography.

The issues of most concern appear to be:

What are the requirements for capturing various types of conventional radiographs
What are the requirements for displaying them for primary and secondary diagnosis
How do certain commercially available systems perform with respect to these criteria
What test procedures can be devised to ensure adequate performance of such systems

An ancillary, but vital question is related to the choice of test data sets. Since the performance required depends on the type (and difficulty) of the clinical material, the choice of test data sets is critical,and presents special problems.

Material

A number of different display systems was tested. In particular, two commercially available systems designed for use as PACS consoleswere investigated. A detailed technical specification of these systems will not be presented here, but it is appropriate to point out that thefirst of these (System 1) included two laser film digitizers (scanning spot size approximately 100 microns), and a display terminal consisting of a 4-monitor viewing station (1024 line monitors, 48MHz band width and 8-bit video coding), with an interlaced display. The second system (System 2) included two laser film digitizers (scanning spot size 200 microns), and a display terminal consisting of 2 monitors (1280 line monitors with a band width corresponding to 70MHz, and12-bit video coding), with a non-interlaced display. In addition three other monitors were tested, the first being a 512x512 display running at 60Hz, the second being 800x600 at 50Hz, and final system being a 640x480 display, running at 50Hz.

The purpose of this paper is not to produce a detailed evaluation of these systems, but to indicate in general what the requirements of a PACS display console are likely to be, and to suggest methods for testing such systems to ensure that their performance is as specified.

Trials were performed to compare physical characteristics that determine image quality for these various monitors functioning at different resolutions. The quality of monitors used in PACS workstations significantly affects the clinical results that can be obtained. However, defining the resolution that would be required for such systems depends critically on the type of clinical data to be interpreted on that system. There is accordingly an interaction between the physical tests and test data sets, and the potential clinical uses of the system.

We also investigated the quality of data acquisition by film digitization,using phantoms and test objects.

Physical Parameters

A number of potential sources of image degradation are listed in Table 1. On the left are shown the more fundamental characteristics, and on the right, the more obvious types of visual effects that they cause.

Table 1

Fundamental Parameters	Effects
Stationarity with position uniformity	Grey level Vignetting Spatial distortion Chances of colour
Stationarity with time	Flicker Jitter Reproducibility of grey scale
Signal to noise ratio	No of grey levels Electronic noise Video line visibility
Transfer function	Resolution Veiling glare Sharpness of edges

In general, although one ideally would wish to quantify the more fundamental parameters, one is constrained to measure the more accessible parameters indicated here as 'effects'. It is also important to note that many of these parameters interact. Thus, for example, signal to noise ratio is significantly effected by flicker.

The performance of the various monitors was evaluated in terms of a number of different parameters: for the purposes of this study, it was considered that the displays could be characterized in terms of:

a) grey level uniformity
b) flicker
c) resolution
d) jitter
e) spatial distortion
and
f) stability with time.

In addition, an attempt was made to measure the stationarity of these properties. By the term 'stationarity' we mean that characteristic of the system relating the performance of the display at different positions across its surface. Therefore, strictly, grey level uniformity is one measure of stationarity, but we can also measure the stationarity of resolution, spatial distortion, etc.

It is known that the eye is very insensitive to certain types of error, for example, variations in grey level across the display. It was however particularly interesting to attempt an objective assessment of flicker and jitter since these appeared to be very disturbing, especially on the display that was used for the ROC tests. By the term 'flicker', we mean those temporal variations in grey level output perceived by the eye at frequencies of 1-100Hz. By the term 'jitter', we mean spatial motion of the displayed image at similar frequencies. Note that most of systems under study were running at 60Hz rather than the normal both 50Hz European standard.

The question of the use of zoom was also of interest. Most systems are capable of some kind of zoom operation whereby part of an image is displayed at a higher resolution than can be used for the whole image. This has been suggested as a method where, for example 2kx2k images, which obviously cannot be displayed at full resolution on any of the systems tested, may be displayed at full resolution, one quadrant at a time. It is not known whether the use of zoom in fact enables the same diagnostic interpretation to be achieved as a higher resolution display capable of showing the whole image in a single frame. This is obviously an important issue with respect to the costs of such systems.

Method

It was considered that the essential measurement to be made was that of light output from the phosphor of the display. The basic method used was to place a fast photodiode (BPX65, Radiospares) looking at light output over small regions. This diode was placed close to the screen, and incorporated a lens in front of the active surface, limiting the area from which light could be detected to a region of about 2mmx2mm (depending on the distance from away from the phosphor). A conventional 100Mhz oscilloscope was used to determine high frequency effects (such as phosphor decay) and a frequency analyzer (HP....) was used to look at low frequency effects, in the region of 5Hz up to 1KHz. More sophisticated devices have been described by other authors. It is also possible to look at the electronic signal being input to the display and to measure such parameters as bandwidth, electronic dynamic width etc. Such experiments are not reported here.

Grey level uniformity was measured by looking at the output from the diode at various positions, and also monitored by using a (slow) light cell based densitometer, also moved manually. An alternative would be to look at the display with an appropriate TV camera system, after corrections for non-uniformity of the camera itself.

Resolution along the video line can be measured by looking at the oscilloscope trace from a single bright dot on the monitor. Resolution is primarily determined by the electronic performance of the display, but also significantly affected by the phosphor temporal and spatial characteristics of the display screen.

Jitter could be determined in part from triggered information observed on the oscilloscope trace, and in part, by visual estimation of displacement looking through a small slit. In the first case, given a high contrast spot, for example part of a ASCII character on the screen, it was possible to trigger the oscilloscope to the signal from one video 'dot'. Frame by frame variations could then be observed. In the second case, by use of the slit and a suitable high contrast detail, the physical shift of the position of the detail across (or down) the screen could be assessed.

Flicker on the other hand is more difficult to measure. What appears to be disturbing are variations in intensity at relatively low frequencies in the region of 1Hz up to 100Hz. These were assessed by looking at the frequency power spectrum. Various other features were observed, in particular, the refresh rate, the interlace (when present) and also interference from 50Hz (mains) frequency which seems to be impossible to eliminate.

The effect of flicker also cannot be easily determined. The visual temporal response is not constant, and certain frequencies can be'inhibited'. However, as is well known the rods do not response to frequencies greater than about 20Hz, while the cones have a higher frequency cut-off. Thus flicker affects particularly the peripheral vision. This is especially troublesome with arrays of monitors in the conventional layout of PACS consoles.

RESULTS: SPECTRUM ANALYSIS

On one particular (60Hz non interlaced) display, the 50Hz peak was very prominent, and (in part) comes from pickup and from the instrumentation itself. A 30Hz peak was visible coming from the interlacing of the display. There was relatively broad spread of the 60Hz peak, with a full width to half maximum of about 5Hz.

On the trace obtained from a better, 60Hz non-interlaced display, the 30Hz peak has disappeared, and the 60Hz peak is much sharper. The broadening of the 60Hz peak was associated with low frequency components in the 1-5Hz range, precisely the low frequency flicker and jitter that we were attempting to measure.

Most of these measurements do not require specialized equipment, and could be performed by a humble microcomputer and ADC connected (after an anti-aliasing filter) to the photodiode.

Tests with a low contrast phantom

A low contrast phantom was designed, being composed of a number of sheets of blank, conventional x-ray film, with holes of different sizes cut from different numbers of sheets, and superimposed. They were radiographed with a variable amount of scattering material present. The phantom presented on a uniform background a number of regions of variable low contrast and different size. The sizes ranges from 6mm down to about 1mm. The addition of different amounts of scatter rendered these lesions more or less difficult to interpret.

A set of 50 films were prepared and then digitized using a laser digitizer at 200 micron scanning spot size. The images were then displayed on the monitor, and the observers asked to record simply how many lesions that though they could observe. The observers were asked to record the same information for the original undigitized films. For each pair of images (digitized and undigitized) the difference between the number of lesions visible was recorded and used in the statistical analysis. These images were interpreted by a total of 6 radiologists.

It is important to note that, on the digitized images, which were essentially uniform, the observers were allowed to use the window functions of the display to enhance the contrast of the image. The main limit to such contrast enhancement was a residual non-uniformity of the digitized film, and the noise of the digitization process. These lesions were in no way limited by spatial resolution. Thus the main purpose of this experiment was to test the noise properties of the digitizer. The results showed that lesion detectability on the monitor was significantly better than on the original film.

A set of physical phantom films has also been proposed, using a high definition photo-typesetter.

Clinical Test Data Sets

Specifically, two types of clinical data sets are required: the first being very demanding, and allowing the performance of the system to be determined for the most difficult types of cases likely to be encountered, and the second being a data set more representative of the routine clinical workload.

Thus, in order to test a system to its limits, it is necessary to choose a pathological condition for study that is subtle, and difficult to diagnose even on film. One series selected was that of subperiosteal resorption in renal osteodystrophy.

A series of 40 hand radiographs was chosen. Half were from patients who had no known renal disease, and who had attended the X-ray department for unrelated conditions; the other half were from patients with proven chronic renal failure in whom a diagnosis of subperiosteal resorption had been evident radiologically on at least two occasions and in whom the diagnosis was also visible to the radiologist administering the tests (RMD); the cases were also shown to radiologists not participating in the study. Patients with obvious metaphyseal changes or other ancillary features were excluded. Some of the cases selected were extremely subtle.

The preliminary findings have been reported elsewhere, but it is clear that there is a significant difference in diagnostic quality between the displayed images and original film. These differences do not appear to be purely a function of matrix size, and may be partly the result of factors such as the physical parameters discussed above.

Further clinical series have been generated using chest radiographs from patients with a pathologically proven diagnosis of Pneumocystis carinii pneumonia, and mammograms from patients with carcinoma of the breast, and additional series of images are also in preparation.

Several important issues are raised. It is clear that a system cannot to tested using only obvious cases; subtle effects must be present, and there must be a significant chance of a feature not being visible: it is necessary to be able to create doubt in the mind of the observer. This necessarily introduces an element of bias. It is possible to use series of images that more closely represent the routine workload, but results in these circumstances would be affected by a priori factors, such as knowledge of the types and incidence of radiological features.

Another issue is that, in order to evaluate such studies, the truth of the observation must be known. This implies either that the evidence for the presence or absence of a feature must be determined from external evidence, or that 'truth' must be established by inspection of the radiological images by some 'higher authority' typically a panel of experts. In the first case, the fact that a feature was not detected must be dangerous. There does not seem to be an ideal solution to this dilemma. Basically, the safest approach seems to be to compare systems using a well validated set of test images, and to perform several trials.

There are further difficulties. ROC studies are normally performed on binary decisions, normal/abnormal, or feature present/absent. However, normal radiological reporting involves making a statement about the image, or (in many cases) making a differential diagnosis, identifying features and indicating their position. Thus not only should one include the ability to localize features, but one should also perform studies where there are multiple, perhaps many, possible decision outcomes. Such data is not easy to analyze, and work is in progress to apply ROC methodology in circumstances that are more representative of the clinical diagnostic process.

Conclusions

The main conclusions that follow from this investigation may be stated as follows:

  1. There are important sources of image degradation

  2. It is important to perform objective tests, such as described, in particular to look at flicker and jitter.

  3. Such tests can be performed using readily available apparatus

If the aim of implementing a PACS system is to be able to perform primary diagnosis on workstations, then it must be stated that this does not yet seem to be achievable on the relatively low resolution monitors that are frequently used and are most widely available. This conclusion applies to the interpretation of subtle effects in conventional radiography, and does not apply to the digital images obtained by CT, MRI etc.

While this conclusion might appear to be a statement of the obvious, such trials need to be performed in order to evaluate the additional cost, complexity, and specification of equipment that would be needed to eliminate the likelihood of mis-diagnosis. It should also be noted that the use of zoom as a device to achieve higher resolution did not achieve much better clinical performance. Thus a further conclusion suggested is that resolution itself (or the lack of it) is not the only source of image degradation of importance.

Further trials of a similar nature, using appropriate data sets, are a necessary part of the process of moving towards the implementation of clinically viable PACS networks.

Acknowledgements

We would like to acknowledge the support of the Department of Health and Social Security, and of Philips Medical Systems, UK.

References

Capp, M P, Roehrig, H, Seeley, G W, Fisher, H D, Ovitt, T W (1985) The digital radiology department of the future. Radiologic Clinics of North America 23, 2 349-354.

Carterette E C, Fiske R A, Huang, H K (1986) Receiver operating characteristic (R O C) evaluation of a digital viewing station for radiologists. S P I E proceedings, 626, 441-446

Craig, J O M C (1988) The filmless department. British journal of hospital medicine. 40, 97-101

Craig, J O M C (1985) Diagnostic radiology without films. The practitioner, 229, 1011-15

Dawood R M, Craig J O M C, Highman J H, Wadsworth J, Glass H I, Todd-Pokropek A, Cunningham D A, Stevens J M, Al-Kutoubi   A, Kerslake R W, Barber C J, Crofton M C, Porter A W (1989).Clinical diagnosis from digital displays: preliminary findings of the St Mary's evaluation project. Clinical radiology, 40, 369-373.

Seeley, G W, Fisher, H D, Stempski, M O, Borgstrom, M, Bjelland, J Capp, M P (1987) Total digital radiology department: spatial resolution requirements.   American journal of roentgenology.148, 421-426.

Specific aspects of compression algorithms for medical imaging

JF. Lerallut, J. Duchene , R. Kanz
Université de Compiègne.Dpt. Génie Biologique, UA CNRS 858
BP 649- 60206 Compiègne Cedex. France

Due to their multiple origins, medical images are very different, not only in terms of resolution (number of pixels) or number of grey levels or colors, but also by the medical and clinical information they hold: a shape, a texture, a contour,etc. Furthermore, the same image may contain different kinds of information for two different specialists, for example one type of information used for diagnosis, and another type for pre-chirurgical purpose. Thus, in a transmission and archiving system,one has to take into account this specificity in order to fit the best compression algorithm with a particular image. Of course, exact coding methods will keep the entire information and reproduce the original image without any degradation, but with a poor compression ratio. Using compression techniques with a loss of information will lead to the determination of what is the "non-interesting" information (for example the background, or the redundancy between adjacent points), and whether the reconstructed image will be as interpretable as the original one by the users. In medicine, the word "interpretable" is related to the visual notion of quality, which is highly subjective and thus can only be qualitative and comparative.

This discrimination between essential and secondary information can be based either on a subjective estimation of quality, like a limited number of grey levels or a lowered resolution, or by means of some statistical criteria such as variance or power contribution. The major problem is to find an acceptability level for this loss of information ,depending on the components of the image itself. Most of the time, the methods used to quantify the difference between original and reconstructed images are statistical (correlation, distance, mse, etc), therefore objective but "blind" . Concerning adaptative algorithms, based on local information of a small area in the image, they do not provide either the same compression factor or the same reconstruction error, depending on the origin of the image.

Without any further decision rules, the best assessment for the choice of a compression method would be, for example, to use a run-length method if the number of grey levels is low, a predictive algorithm if the dynamic range is poor, some kind of low-pass filtering if the useful information is the general aspect of the image ,or on the opposite a high frequency enhancement if only the borders of objects or their number are of any interest. Most of the time a hybrid combination of several algorithms will give the best results, in terms of compression efficiency and noticeable degradation.

Another way for coding is to use an exact compression method in a region of interest with maximum resolution, thus avoiding any loss of information in this area, and to use a more powerful algorithm in terms of compression ratio but with a lower quality of reconstruction in all other parts of the image, like the background.

Then the problem is to extract those regions of interest, according to criteria that could only be defined by medical experts for each of the considered applications. For example, the discrimination between pertinent information and uninteresting background is easier to perform on some echographies or bone X-rays or RMN images than on pulmonary X-rays or in quantitative microscopy and histologic images.

In order to perform this expertise, a set of reference images should be settled, covering the multimedia aspects of medical imaging for efficient and reliable archiving and transmission. From this set, a strategy could be derived to fit the best compression algorithm for each class of images.

References

1) Bernard M., Kunt M., Leonardi R., Volet P.:"Analyse de scènes et compression d'images".*BULL. SEV /VSE* 77 - première partie 1986;.11: n°7,pp 621-631 - deuxième partie 1986;21:n°8, pp 1373-1379

2) Chen W., Pratt W.K.:"Scene adaptative coder" . IEEE Trans. Commun.1984; COM-32;n°3, pp 225-232,

3) Huang H.K., Lo S.C., Ho B.K., Lou S.L. :"Radiological image compression using error-free and irreversible two-dimensional direct cosine transform coding techniques" *J. Opt. Soc. Am.* .1987;4,pp 984-992

4) Hubel D.H., Wiesel T.:"Brain mechanism of vision", *Scien. Am.*, 1979 ;.241, n°3, pp 150-162.

5) Jain A.K.: "Image data compression : a review", *Proc. IEEE*, 1981; 69:pp 349-389

6) Kunt M.:" Source coding of X-ray pictures", *IEEE Trans. on Biomed.Eng..* 1978;Vol.BME-25,pp 121-138.

7) Metz C.E.:" Basic principles of ROC analysis". *Sem. in Nucl. Med..*1978; 8: n° 4,pp 283-298.

8) Netravali A.N., Limb J.:" Picture coding : a review".*Proc. IEEE*, 1980;.68,pp 366-406.

9) Noh. K.H., Jenkins J.M.:" Comparision of data compression schemes for medical images. Application of optical instrumentation in medicine and Picture archiving and communication systems (PACS IV)". Schneider and Dwyer eds., *SPIE* . 1986;.626, pp 392-398.

10) Peters J.H., Roos P., Van Dijke M.C., Viergever M.A., Loss-less: "Compression in digital angiography. Information Processing in Medical Imaging." De Graff and Viergever eds., *Plenum Press.* 1987: pp 335-341

Caracterisation et classification des images médicales en vue d'une compression optimale.

R. Kanz* **
* Laboratoire de Biomécanique et Instrumentation médical / UA 858 CNRS Université de Technologie de Compiègne / France
** Laboratoire de Microélectronique Appliquée Centre de Recherche Public - Henri Tudor. Luxembourg

Cet article propose une nouvelle méthodologie dont le but est la détermination de l'algorithme de compression d'images optimal, par un système de décision basé sur une caractérisation et classification des images médicales en fonction de leurs propriétés texturales. Ce système de décision est réalisé grâce à une "pyramide discriminante", basée sur des analyses factorielles discriminantes successives.

We suggest in this paper a new methodology which consists in choosing the optimal encoding algorithm by an expert system based on a characterization and classification of medical images by means of textural characteristics. This expert system is constructed by means of a "discriminant pyramid", which is based on successive discriminating Karhunen-Loeve classifications.

1. Introduction

Les images médicales sont issues de sources de plus en plus diversifiées, et les examens qui y correspondent sont de plus en plus nombreux et complexes.

Cette augmentation importante de la masse d'informations disponibles pose aux centres hospitaliers de nouveaux problèmes de transfert et d'archivage. Ces problèmes sont actuellement traités de façon ponctuelle, grâce à des algorithmes de compression qui sont à usage général et donc dans de nombreux cas inadaptés à l'imagerie médicale, en terme d'efficacité.

Indépendamment des supports qui vont se développer, il est important d'aborder l'archivage et le transfert des images médicales en développant non seulement des algorithmes de compression, mais également des méthodes de choix optimal de l'un ou l'autre d'entre eux en fonction de la caractéristique de l'image.

2. Methodes d'analyse de la texture

La méthode des *matrices de cooccurrence* (4) consiste à caractériser les images en fonction de la dépendance spatiale existante au niveau des valeurs de gris de différents pixels.
Les quatre matrices reflètent la dépendance dans les directions de O°, 45°, 90° et 135° degrés et décrivent finalement les probabilités de transition. Ensuite on peut à partir de ces matrices calculer des paramètres reflétant le contraste, la corrélation, la variance et bien d'autres paramètres.
Une autre méthode intéressante est celle du *vecteur des différences de niveaux de gris.* (10). Elle utilise des statistiques sur les propriétés locales différentielles d'ordre 1, en formant les

différences absolues entre les niveaux de gris adjacents et selon de nouveau quatre directions.

A partir du vecteur des différences possibles, nous pouvons calculer les indices tel que le contraste, l'entropie,....

Les histogrammes directionnels (9), basés sur la caractéristique vectorielle du gradient permettent de voir s'il y a par exemple des directions privilégiées dans l'image.

Une autre méthode est basée sur le calcul des *plages* (4) d'un même niveau de gris dans les quatre directions.

Il existe même des techniques basées sur le calcul d'un modèle autoregressif pour décrire l'image (4).

3. Methodologie adoptée pour la construction du système de décision

Se rendant compte que les méthodes de compression d'images sont sensibles à des propriétés spécifiques de l'image et impliquant en fonction de ces propriétés des résultats de codage variables, il est intéressant de mettre en évidence la relation existante entre les caractéristiques texturales de l'image et les résultats obtenus en fonction d'un type de compression.

Dans un premier temps il est important de définir différentes classes d'images médicales par des méthodes d'analyse factorielle (3) (5) et d'analyser les résultats de différents algorithmes sur les images compressées. De même il faut définir l'erreur relative maximale qui peut être induite par la compression en relation avec les experts concernés en particulier les radiologues.
Ceci représente la phase d'apprentissage du système.

Dans un deuxième temps sera créé une "pyramide discriminate" dont la base représente la totalité des classes d'images possibles. Les plans discriminants successifs de la pyramide décrivent des classes de plus en plus précises.

Ainsi en effectuant une classification en cascade de l'image dans la pyramide discriminante nous arrivons à un niveau (sommet) ou chaque classe correspond à un algorithme de compression le mieux adapté (voir fig. 1).

4.   Premiers résultats

Dans une première étude de caractérisation d'images médicales a été utilisé un vecteur paramétrique se composant d'indices obtenus à partir de la méthode des différences de niveaux de gris et de l'histogramme directionnel.

Ensuite ont été calculés les indices de texture pour une population d'images médicales de types différents telque des échographies, des images scanner, des angiographies, images I.R.M.

Le vecteur final paramétrisant une image se compose des éléments suivants:

1. Contraste*
2. Moment angulaire d'ordre 2*
3. Entropie*
4. Moyenne*
5. Première direction privilégiée**
6. Deuxième direction privilégiée**

Nous avons effectué une analyse factorielle discriminante sur la population de tous les vecteurs paramétriques représentant nos images (calcul des deux premiers facteurs).

Dans la fig. 2 et fig. 3 nous montrons les résultat obtenus pour la discrimination de classes entre des images de type :

1. scanner / I.R.M.
2. échographie / scanner

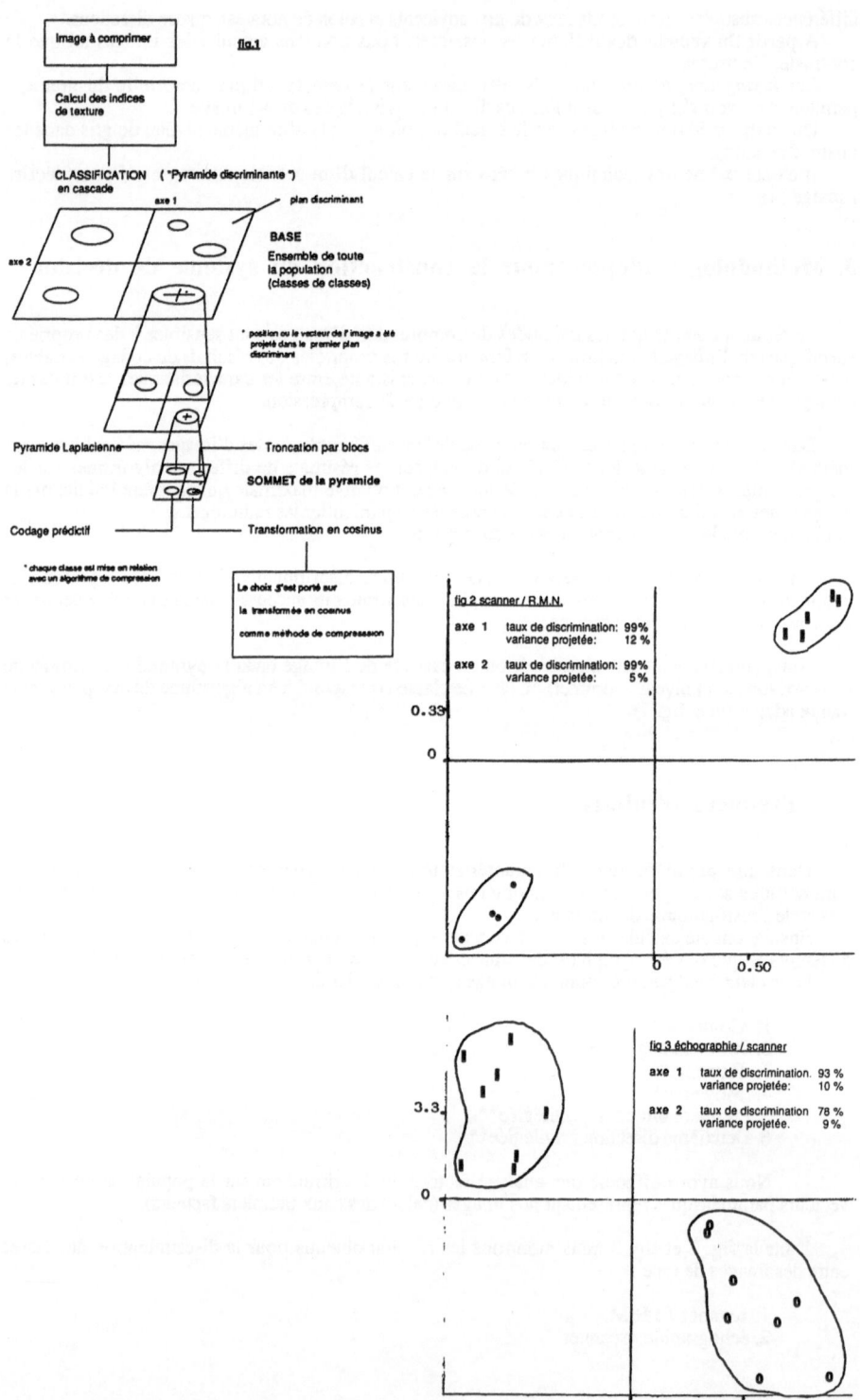

fig.1

Image à comprimer

Calcul des indices de texture

CLASSIFICATION ("Pyramide discriminante ")
en cascade

axe 1   plan discriminant

axe 2

BASE
Ensemble de toute
la population
(classes de classes)

* position ou le vecteur de l'image a été
projeté dans le premier plan
discriminant

Pyramide Laplacienne   Troncation par blocs

SOMMET de la pyramide

Codage prédictif   Transformation en cosinus

* chaque classe est mise en relation
avec un algorithme de compression

Le choix s'est porté sur
la transformée en cosinus
comme méthode de compression

fig 2 scanner / R.M.N.

axe 1   taux de discrimination: 99%
         variance projetée: 12 %

axe 2   taux de discrimination: 99%
         variance projetée: 5 %

0.39

0

0   0.50

fig 3 échographie / scanner

axe 1   taux de discrimination. 93 %
         variance projetée: 10 %

axe 2   taux de discrimination   78 %
         variance projetée.   9 %

3.3

0

0   0.63

On voit par les métodes de paramétrisation et de classification choisies que l'on obtient des résultats intéressants (Taux de discrimination supérieur à 93 %).

De même on a pu montrer une bonne stabilité des classes trouvées, par les méthodes des "nuées dynamiques" ou des "kppv".

6. Conclusion

Pour cette étude les images ont d'abord été caractérisées d'après leurs composantes texturales. Pour cela il a fallu définir un vecteur paramétrique composé d'indices de texture obtenus à partir des vecteurs de différence de gris et de l'histogramme directionnel. Ces vecteurs ont été calculés pour plusieurs types d'images médicales (I.R.M., échographies, scanner, etc...).Utilisée en référence de manière à valider la méthode de caractérisation, une analyse factorielle discriminante a permis de mettre en évidence la capacité de ce système de paramètres à séparer correctement les différentes classes d'images. A chaque classe correspond un algorithme de compression différent, choisi en fonction du taux et de l'erreur de compression obtenus. Les premiers résultats montrent qu'il est possible d'appliquer à une image donnée l'algorithme de compression le mieux adapté, en utilisant une combinaison des différents paramètres de texture.

REFERENCES

1. **M. Bernard, M. Kunt, R. Leonardi, P. Volet,** "Analyse des scènes et compression d'images" BULL. SEV / VSE77,- première parie Vol. 11 n°7 juin   1986   pp 621-631- deuxième partie Vol. 21 n)8 novembre 1986 pp 1373 -1379

2. **R. J. Clarke,** "Transform coding of image", Microelectronics and signal processing,Academic Press 1985

3. **J. Duchène,** "Développement de méthodes de décision sur un ensemble de   tableaux", Thèse de doctorat d'Etat, Université de Technologie de Compiègne   1983

4. **L. van Gool, P. Dewaele, A. Oosterlink,** "Texture analysis anno 1983",   Computer vision, graphics and image proc.Academic Press, Vol. 29 1985

5. **L. Lebart, A. Morineau, J.P. Fenelon,**" Traitement des données   statistiques",Dunod 1982

6. **A.N. Netravali, B.G. Haskell,**"Digital Pictures", Plenum Press,1988

7. **W.K. Pratt,**"Digital Image Processing",John Wiley and Sons New York 1987

8. **À. Rosenfeld, A. C. Kak,**"Digital Picture Processing", Vol.   1,Academic Pres,1982

9. **H. Tamura, S. Mori, T.Yamawarki** "Texture features corresponding to visual perception", IEEE Trans. on syst., man   and Cybernetics,Vol. SMC-8, n°6 june 1978 pp 460-473

10. **J.S. Weszka, C.R.Dyer, A. Rosenfeld,**"A comparative study of texture measures for terrain classificaton",IEEE Tranf. on syst., man and cybernetics,Vol.   SNC-6, n°4 april 1076,pp 269-285

Differentiation and Requirements of Image-computers in a Clinical PACS Environment

R. Mattheus, R. Van den Broeck, M. Osteaux
Pluridisciplinary Research Institute for Medical Imaging Sciences (PRIMIS)
University Hospital Brussels - Department of Radiology
Laarbeeklaan 101 - B 1090 Brussels, Belgium

For PACS environments in clinical use different classes of requirement-levels for image manipulation and viewing can be defined from a medical, organizational, technical and economical point of view. These requirements have a direct impact on the specifications and cost of the image-computers as well as on their level of integration in the PACS, RIS (Radiology Information System) and HIS (Hospital Information System) environments. Digital imaging used in radiology requires a high quality display console for the medical specialists to review and manipulate images.
This paper aims to give an overview of the classes and requirements of different image-computers used in a clinical environment .

1 Introduction

In 1986 the PACS project at the university hospital of Brussels (VUB), which is a 700 bed teaching hospital started. A part of the PACS realizations are in clinical use since 1989. The main goal of the project was making PACS-units at sub-departments for use in clinical routine. The project focused on two main topics where focused: networking and display techniques.

Digital images can be viewed in two ways : directly on a cathode ray tube (CRT) screen or on photographic film. The design requirements placed on a viewing system are quite stringent if the quality of the system is to approach that of photographic film. These requirements are the most demanding in digital radiology, in which spatial resolution requirements are frequently very high, and least demanding in nuclear medicine, in which spatial resolution is low.

Image-computers used in networks must cope with certain problems not present when an image from only one modality is displayed. The viewing devices must be able to display images having different spatial and contrast resolutions. Furthermore, each type of examination has its own unique requirements for interactive display. The computer associated with the viewing node must allow for the appropriate manipulation and simultaneous display of different kinds of information such as images, acquisition parameters and patient data. The growing availability of digital images has led to the introduction of a wide variety of display stations to be used to present digital radiographic images to the physician.

2 Data Organization

2.1 Introduction

Before handling these enormous amounts of information (display, storing and manipulation) a structure for organizing these data, based on the medical relevance is defined. An examination type is defined as a 8-tuple, which gives us a platform for calculations of the amount of data to be handled.

2.2 Information structure

In collaboration with Siemens, the hospital in Graz (Vienna) and Victoria hospital (Canada), a concept for the organization of the information and the reduction of the amount of data has been developed [1]. One of the fundamental considerations was not to cast away any digital image generated. Therefore those images which are not relevant for the diagnosis, are reduced to a 128x128 / 8 bit image (overview). Images selected by the radiologist are kept in full matrix size.

Actual examination folder (AEF) :
This folder contains all images of the actual examination including reformatted images at full

size. In addition to each image a 128x128 pixel image is created to be displayed in the overview image. During the interpretation and reporting of the study, relevant images can be marked for archiving in full resolution.

Final Examination Folder (FEF) :
In this folder all images of the examination are present as token images. The relevant images, which have been marked during reporting are available in the original matrix. Only those images can be selected and displayed in full resolution.

Hospitalization Report Folder (HRF) :
In the HRF all FEF's of one patient are included. This folder is the image-medical record of the patient. All the images are in this folder.

Special Examination Folder (SEF) :
This folder contains various collections of selected images (e.g. private collection for the radiologist) for teaching and scientific purposes. Images of different patients can be put together.

Final Review Examination Folder (FREF) :
The radiologist can mark images, which can be reviewed by the clinicians. For these selected images the gray-level scale (contrast resolution) is reduced to the most significant part. This reduces the amount of data with 50%.

2.3 Examination type

Images are central objects in a medical environment. For PACS it is important to consider a group of images as one identity. A clinician will look at an examination of a patient, which consists of several images. This group of images can be described by 8 parameters. Based on this 8-tuple, minimum requirements can be calculated for image-computers (resolution manipulation functions, storage).

Definition of a 8-tuple (M,E,N,S,R,D,T,C) : Examination type
- M : {CT,MR,US,DR,XR,DSA} modality source
- E : {body, head, neuro, cardiac, abdominal, vasc, bone} examination
- N : maximum number of images
- S : maximum number of marked images
- R : {64,128,256,512,1024,2048,4096} matrix n.n
- D : {2,3,4} display technique (depends on acquisition)
  - 2 : 2D image (x,y)
  - 3 : image of a 3D set(x,y,z)
  - 4 : image in a dynamic 3D set (x,y,z,t)
- T : average examination time
- C : {8,12} contrast resolution in grey level

M	E	N	S	R	D	T	C	class
CT	Body	34	21	512	2	30	12	A
	Head	20	15	512	2	30	12	A
MR	Body	80	13	256	2	40	12	A
	Neuro	128	13	256	3	40	12	E
	Bone	173	25	256	3	55	12	E
	Cardio	19	19	256	4	35	12	C
US	Body	8	4	512	2	20	8	A
DR	Body	8	8	4096	2	15	12	B
DSA	Cardio	400	20	512	4	20	12	C
	Cardio	100	20	1024	4	30	12	C
	Vasc	400	20	512	4	30	12	C
PET	Neuro	20	5	256	2	40	8	D
	Cardio	20	5	256	2	40	8	D

Table 1.
Parameters for 8-tuple of the Radiology dep. of the University of Brussels (VUB) 1989.

Five main display classes can be defined (Table 1). Each class has it own hard- and software needs for displaying the examinations depending on (r,d) and the image-computer classes described in section 4.

3 IMAGE-COMPUTERS

3.1 Introduction
An image-computer can be described by three components:
-The internal communications, which are the nerves of the system
The communication with other environments can be described as:
- interaction with the doctors: the user-communication.
- interaction with the network and other systems: the external communication.

3.2 Definition of digital images
An image can be defined in terms of its actual information or by the maximum information which could be contained in its space. The TV bandwidth is the electrical bandwidth required to carry the information (function of limiting resolution, frame rate, number of scanning lines / frame). The information content is the effective total maximum possible information of a single frame (dimensions, S/N). The digital content is the digital value of information in function of the digital value of the number of pixels. Images can be quantized by the scanning process or by the nature of the detectors, e.g. a matrix of cells as in the case of CCD's [2].

3.3 Architecture of image computers

3.3.1 Internal communication
An attribute which impacts the quality of a medical imaging workstation is the performance of the system. Radiologists see the performance of image-computers through the amount of time that the system takes to display or manipulate the image on the screen. Tasks done by the software can be executed by the general workstation processor or by a graphics processing unit.

A graphics accelerator provides specialised hardware to perform operations on images and data on the workstation (e.g. zoom, inverse, rotate).

3.3.2 User - communication
Display
The most important attribute of the display is the resolution of the displayed image. The resolution consists of two parameters. First, the number of pixels on the screen determines the amount of information that the image can contain, *the spatial resolution* . Second the number of bits to represent each pixel is important for the *contrast resolution*. The number of gray levels is limited to 2 to the power of the number of bits used(12 bit- 4069 gray levels).
Images constructed by an acquisition modality consist of information that is made available by the physical principle used by that particular modality. The image presentation is a modification of these constructed images. Different variables will have an influence on that modification e.g.: spatial resolution, contrast resolution, display flicker and post processing. Some variables are related to the observer, such as environmental conditions (light), psychological factor and age. Most of the images (99%) are gray-level images, representing morphological information; colour is only used for functional information such as blood flow (when using colour for morphological information, false contours could appear when moving from one colour to another).

Image presentation
   - same as standard film
   - minimal delay
   - limited number of monitors
   - high refresh rate

High Definition TV
In comparison with conventional television, HDTV offers extremely clear images. The currently used NTSC-PAL standards employs 525-625 lines. HDTV has 1125 lines. The resulting picture is equivalent to that obtained with 35mm motion picture film. A second difference is the aspect ratio of the HDTV screen which is 16:9 in contrast to 4:3 ratio. The result is a magnificent feeling of nearness. The viewing distance is three times the screen height. As a system

for display purposes HDTV is expected to find wide applications in every branch of medical science.

<u>User-interface</u>
    The user interface plays an important role in the success of a PACS application. It is essential that a close interaction exists between the designers and the users.
The different forms of interactive man-machine dialogue can be classified in 3 major categories :

    -user driven dialogue based on a command language.
    -system driven dialogue: the user answers the questions presented by the system filling forms
      or selecting menu items
    -direct manipulation: the user tells to the system the actions which must be performed e.g.
      Apple Macintosh

Interactive functions
    - Simple
    - Menu driven
    - logical function organization
    - limited functions for image processing

    In a PACS environment, the screen should be free to display a large number of images. Therefore, menus should be kept as small as possible. However, the image manipulation command style should match some complex actions not easily described. To solve these design challenges and provide users with flexible, customised products, specific software components are necessary. X-windows is an example of a software tool for the development of user-interfaces.
    When using X-windows portability is ensured because of the open character of its conception. X/Open represents a major breakthrough in the world of Open Systems. X/Open is not a standard-setting body. It is a joint initiative by members of the business community to adapt existing standards into a consistent environment.

<u>Devices for user interaction</u>
    Although alphanumeric keyboards are still very important in computer applications, they need to be avoided. Additional devices must be used to interact with imaging applications: mouses and trackballs are used to point at selected areas of the images or operate "iconic" commands.
    Digitizing tables offer more accurate guidance for selecting a region of interest in the display. Rotating knobs, function keys can be designed to enhance ergonomy (center-windowing). Voice interaction will become important, when it also will be used for digital voice storage (reporting).

3.3.3   External communication
    External communication of an image-computer is one of the most critical factors because the lack of standards.[3]
    External communication has three main components.
    - hardware interface.
    - commands.
    - data-formats.
    The American College of Radiology (ACR), representing the users of imaging equipment, and the National Electrical Manufacturers Association (NEMA), representing the manufactures of imaging equipment, joined forces to address the issues involving compatibility in electronic exchange of digital medical images[4]. A few standard are defined and become available on hardware level first published in 1985. SPI (Standard Product Interconnect), a joint effort of Siemens and Philips, which is a partial extension of the ACR/NEMA format is implemeted by Siemens in its new products. A fundamental premise in SPI is that each modality is allowed to retain as much autonomy as possible, consistent with overall system integrity requirements.
    The goals of the open imaging systems architecture include the following:
- Provide a consistent basis for conceptual communication among system designers regarding imaging systems.
- Define a generic operating environment over a wide range of hardware and software imaging components.

4 Classes of Imaging Computers

4.1 Introduction
Various image-computers are required to obtain an effective PACS. Two main types can be considered:
- Image/data acquisition (Input)
    - Film input
    - Data input
- Image display stations (Output)
    - Specialized image stations (SIS)
    - Images processing station (IPS)
    - Multi modality reporting console (MRC)
    - Multi modality viewing station (MVS)
    - Remote viewing Station (RVS)
    - Multi modality film output (MF)

4.2 Specialized image stations (SIS)
A specialized image station forms the interface between an acquisition unit, and the medical and technical user. The hard- and software of these stations is dedicated to each type of acquisition modality (CT, MRI). This console belongs to the acquisition unit and allows the processing of the raw data and image manipulations. It must also provides the possibility to make the image available in the PACS environment.

Three main problems appear for integration in a PACS environment.

First, images are in the format of the modality (company and modality dependent). Hopefully the ACR/NEMA format will soon be commercially available. Second, patient information (patient id, patient name) is added on this level to the images, with the necessary problems of inconsistent PACS and HIS/RIS DB (mistyping).

Thirdly, the acquisition unit is not developed towards integration in a network structure (user-interface, security, system organisation).

sc_{sis}: storage capacity SIS for one modality type (disk)

$$4n(r^2/10^6)*exa\_day = sc_{sis} \text{ Mbyte (1)}$$

exa_day:examinations a day

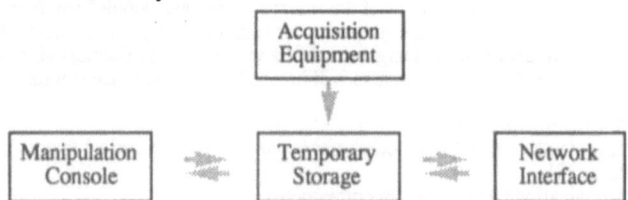

fig 1.

Logical image-flow (fig 1): Information is acquired, calculated and stored on temporary storage medium (1). The stored images can be retrieved and/or processed on the SIS, network access to the disk must be possible.

4.3 Image processing stations (IPS)
Function : image processing and manipulation

These stations allow advanced processing applications, unavailable in the specialized image station or common to different modalities, to be implemented more efficiently on a multimodality image processing station.

Such a station requires a large image memory (2), a fast array processor, flexible software and programming tools. It permits detailed investigation and evaluation of 3-D images. It provides the possibility to perform sophisticated manipulations of previously calculated images and is intended for use by the diagnostic imaging specialist.

msc_{ips}: min storage capacity for IPS for one examination type (image ram)

$$3nr^2/10^6 = msc_{ips} \text{ Mbyte (2)}$$

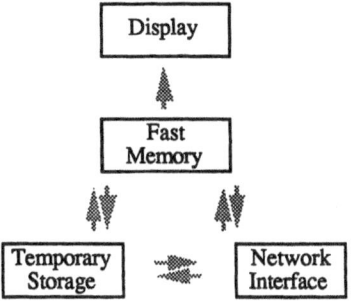

fig 2.

Logical image-flow (fig 2): Direct access between network interface and fast internal memory, which is necessary for high quantity of images.

The IPS should have multiple levels of user interaction,.so that it can be used by people with different backgrounds (engineers, specialists, clinicians, programmers).

- Specific selection of programs
    3D reconstruction
    CAD/CAM prothesis
    flow manipulation
    3D view
- Interactive image processing
- Programming environment
- Array processor programming

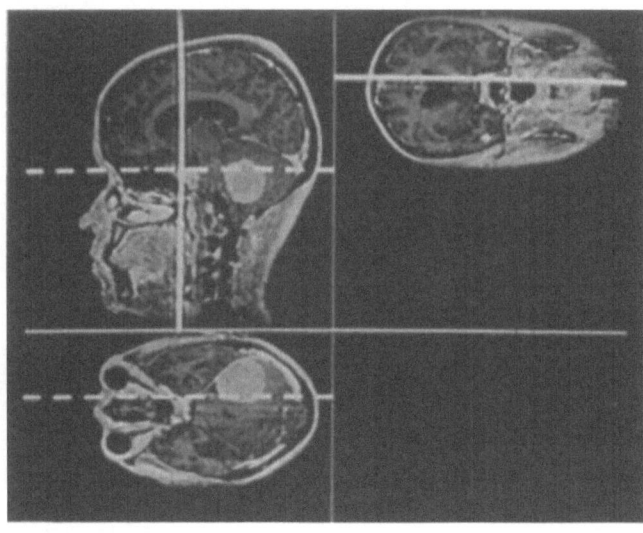

A set of 128 MRI images, calculated on a Kontron IPS.

Requirements for integration IPS

- flexible and easy to use
- dedicated programs
- extensive image processing tools
- large RAM
- fast array processor
- easy to integrate in a network structure
- fast image transfer
- integration with hardcopy unit
- different display possibilities

4.4 Multimodality reporting console (MRC)

Function : interpreting and reporting of examinations

This is the PACS-console. Two types of stations : "multiple" (MRCM) and "virtual" (MRCV) display stations can be considered.

A multiple display station must be capable of displaying several images simultaneously on different image monitors. Instant transfer of images from monitor to monitors allows convenient side-by-side comparisons and some simple low-level image operations.

A virtual display unit uses panning and scrolling in a large image memory to obtain analogous capabilities with a single monitor. The idea of the virtual image station is to roam the images on the screen the same way you do with a microfilm, but instead of moving the head to the left and right, you move the image memory mapping and look at one monitor. This type of reporting can speed up the examination because there is no waiting time after selecting a patient. Both implementations mentioned above are in fact electronic simulations of the arrangement of the conventional films.

msc_{mrc} : minimum storage capacity MRC for one examination type (disk)

$$exa\_day \ (n + s) \ 4r^2/10^6 = msc_{mrc} Mbyte \ (3)$$

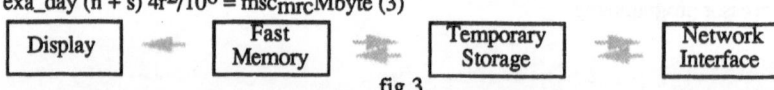

fig 3.

Logical image-flow (Fig3.): Access between network interface and temporary memory.

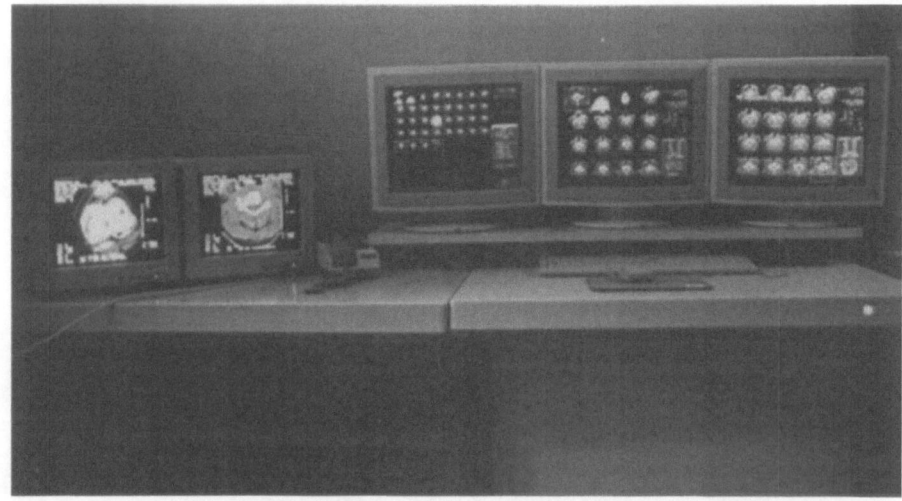

MRC at the CT-PACS reporting section of the university hospital of Brussels (VUB). At the left, two real-time monitors for communication with the two CT- rooms are installed. The MRC is a 3 screen 1kx1k prototype console from Siemens.

Requirements for integration MRC.

- modular design (1 to n high resolution monitors)
- display and individual image processing on each screen
- simultaneous display facilities of digital systems
- text annotation
- compression/decompression
- fast access to the archive
- networking capabilities
- graphic editing (ROI; annotations)
- reporting tools
- contrast modification
- spatial frequency
- user friendly interface

4.5   Multimodality Viewing Station - MVS
Functions: Review of reported images
This type of workstation offers any authorized clinician the possibility to have a quick review of a
patient study. It should be a cheap entry to the PACS environment, with a reduced image set and
good spatial resolution. Only a few image manipulation functions are required. This user-friendly
station must also have the possibility displaying images and reports.

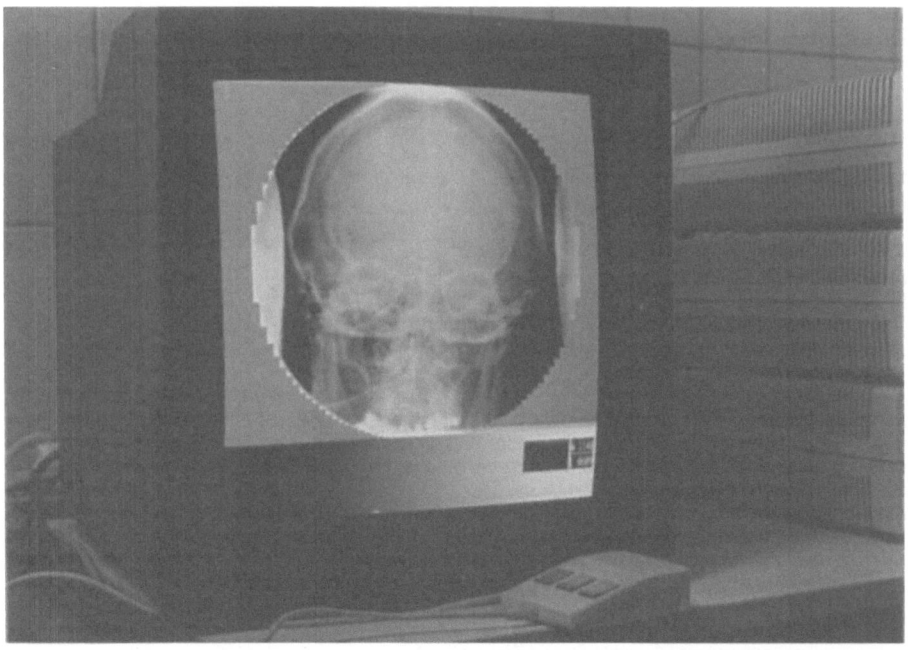

The Imlogix MVS installed at the emergency department at the university hospital of Brussels
(VUB). This station is a 1kx1k, 12 bit directly connected to the ethernet.

Requirements for integration MVS.

- simple to use
- not expensive
- image manipulation tools
        window centre

- report (RIS) / image integration
- fast access to reduced image set
- good spatial resolution

To overcome the display technology barrier, the review console was designed to keep larger images in memory and to display them at a lower resolution. In this unit there is no image buffer available (3). An image server is implemented on a macintosh computer. Pan and zoom functions were built onto the console to allow the user to look at certain sections of the image at full resolution.

msc_{mvs} : minimum storage capacity MVS for one examination type (disk)
exa_day (s) $4r^2/10^6 = msc_{mvs}$ Mbyte (3)

4.6   Remote Viewing Station - RVS
Functions: Review of reported images at remote sides and scientific archive images.

Requirements for integration MVS.

- teleradiology inside / outside the hospital
- telemedecine
- teaching rooms
- simple to use
- not expensive
- image manipulation tools
        window centre
                width
- fast access to reduced image set
- good spatial resolution

msc_{rvs} : minimum storage capacity RVS for one examination type (disk)
exa_day (s) $2r^2/10^6 = msc_{rvs}$ Mbyte (3)

4.7 Multimodality Hardcopy Output - MH
Functions :
Printout of images:
        mixed different modalities (CT,MR,US,...)
        time mode (old and new images)
        patient history (selected images)

In a classic radiology department hardcopy units are directly connected to the modality by video or digital connection. In a PACS environment it is very useful to connect a hardcopy unit to the network in a digital way, so they can used as back-up unit for each other.

Requirements for integration MH.
        workstation driven
        network driven
        - all images
        - selected images
   -    easy and intuitive access to images and patient records
   -    concurrent view of exams from different modalities
   -    support for the report generation process

5   Conclusion
In a PACS environment there will be different classes of images-computers hopeful with the same user-interface, but adapted to the users, their needs and applications. At the moment one of the main problems is that image-computers are developed as stand-alone units. For clinical use fast access to the images is important. For handling this enormous amount of data, large and fast image memory is important. Network management and display techniques will be the key components in new pacs developments.[5]

6 References

1) Greinacher at al.:"System Architecture and Functionality of Structured Siemens PACS *Proc of the V. Isprad* . 1988, p.217.

2).Eastgate, Siedband, Ergun et al.:"A method for evaluation of screen-film combination" *SPIE* 1990;

3) Mattheus, Luypaert, Osteaux, Temmerman: "Hard-and software for integrating special applications in a PACS environment" *.Proc MIE88* (Oslo).Springer-Verlag; 1988; 35.

4).Wang, Best, Hoffman, Horii.et al :"ACR-NEMA Digital Imaging and Communication Standards: Minimum Requirements" *.Radiology* 1988;166:529-532.

5) Jost, Wessell , Blaine et al.:"PACS - Is there light at the end of the tunnel". *SPIE* 1989; 1093 pp74-83

Overview of Video Transmission Activity

A. Pimenta Alves
Universidade do Porto/INESC - Largo Mompilher, 22 - P- 4000 Porto

1 Introduction

The increase in the capacity of modern communication networks, particularly after the introduction of the optical fibre technology, is creating a growing interest in the use of digital techniques for the transmission of images, including moving images that require very high transmission bandwidth. The analogue techniques sometimes used until now for such applications, due to their lower cost, besides the well known disadvantages relative to their digital counterparts, do not allow a convenient integration with other services in a common communication network.

In fact one fundamental characteristic of the foreseen evolution in communication networks is that of total service integration.

In order to reduce to reasonable values the large amounts of data otherwise required by the digital video transmission, different types of compression algorithms are used, according to the quality requirements of each application.

In the following present trends in terms of quality, coding and relevant network aspects are described not only in relation to the transmission in the public network but also in private networks.

Reference will also be made to recent advances in terms of picture coding and coding for the storage and retrieval of moving image and sound in digital storage media. These developments are so important that will have strong impact on all image transmission activities.

In conclusion a short reference is made to related work in progress at INESC.

2 Quality of Digital Video Services

The digital video services normally referred, in order of increasing bandwidth requirements, are videophone, video conference, standard broadcast TV and High Definition TV (HDTV), (Enhanced and Extended Definition TV are considered intermediate steps).

These services were not designed directly aiming at medical applications but it will certainly be possible to find areas of direct application. The advantage of using telecommunication standards will be a significant price reduction and easier supply. However, when discussing PACS in medical environments one should analyse in more detail some other important image handling applications like surveillance image, video sequence data bases, and colour picture storage and retrieval.

Quality requirements for each of these applications together with coder and transmission costs have determined the necessary bit rates for each of these applications.

In spite of the progress recently made in the area there are very few standards approved as a result of certain technological limitations. Hardware limits the possibilities of using complex algorithms particularly in high quality codecs. VLSI is extensively used and codecs are complex and expensive, with costs dropping only when massive production is reached.

Until very recently, due to the characteristics of all existing communication networks, all coding algorithms aimed at a fixed transmission rate therefore introducing variations in the image quality, whenever the information contents of the video sequences was too high to fit in the available bandwidth, and the available compensation buffers were filled.

The detailed analysis of the coding techniques used in this context is out of the scope of this paper. A brief description of the main techniques involved and of some major steps is given below.

Digital TV to be used within studios is already standardized. The adoption of the Rec. 601 from CCIR is considered a significant progress in this area. Its main properties are: it is based on component coding, it creates an extensive family of compatible standards and it is world-wide accepted. The main technical features are:

Sampling Frequency:
> Luminance:13.5 MHz Colour Differences (Cr, Cb): 6.75MHz

Samples per line (625/50 systems):
> Luminance: 864 Colour Differences: 432

Samples per active line:
> Luminance: 720 Colour Differences: 360

Interfaces for studio use were also defined in Rec. 656 from CCIR. The parallel interface, in particular, is well used; it specifies a parallel output at 27Mbyte/s, not allowing long distance transmission.

This Recommendation generates a level of quality that is better than broadcast quality and, because there is no compression, it is very appropriate to allow required image processing, without any further degradation. Whenever possible, this standard or compatible extension should be used in the A/D and D/A components of all image systems.

In terms of long distance transmission the situation is not as advanced. There is presently a considerable activity at all levels aiming at the standardization of various services.

One of the most efficient coding techniques is interframe prediction or motion compensated prediction with conditional picture element replenishment. In these techniques one frame is compared with the previous one and, information is only sent regarding those points or regions in which there is a difference larger than a certain threshold. These methods are obviously appropriate for those situations where there is limited movement in the scene, as it is the case in videophone and teleconference.

Another very efficient technique uses image transforms. One important example is the Discrete Cosine Transform (DCT). Transforms can be used to highly compress image data with very good quality. For reduced bit rates it is normally combined with interframe prediction or motion compensation techniques, to give what is normally designated hybrid coding. The picture is divided in blocks and only the difference towards the predicted block is sent.

Recently, another technique named Vector Quantization, is being explored. In this method picture elements are expressed as vectors and quantized in order to reduce the overall bit rate. This method can be combined with those previously described in order to achieve the higher compression rates.

For higher quality coding the difficulties of implementation limit the use of interframe algorithms. Intraframe algorithms and particularly those implying smaller processing and storage requirements are favoured.

One technique well known is the DPCM, in which a prediction of the current picture sample is obtained using previously coded samples. The prediction error only, after being quantized and coded, is transmitted.

There are a number of variations of this technique described in the literature, some of them using prediction based on interframe samples. However the most interesting techniques for high quality applications use only intraframe prediction. The simplest being the one using a one-dimensional prediction algorithm (prediction within the same line).

The main problem with DPCM techniques is their sensitivity to channel errors. To reduce this sensitivity hybrid PCM/DPCM coding is used, in which PCM coded samples are periodically sent.

A detailed analysis of all these and other algorithms and results of some concrete implementations can be found in the literature [1,2,3,4,5,6,7]. The analysis of the results obtained points towards the following bit rates for the main services discussed:

HDTV   120-140Mbit/s
Standard TV
    Contribution   70-140Mbit/s
    Distribution   15-34Mbit/s
Videoconference   384-2048Kbit/s
Videophone   56-64kbit/s.

There is presently a standard for videoconference at 2Mbit/s. Standardization activity is in progress for a px64kbit/s video-phone/conference codec (p=1 to 30) and for a TV distribution quality codec at 34Mbit/s.

There is however a very important step in the evolution of communication networks taking place now, that will have strong impact on video coding. This is the use of ATM in the future Broadband ISDN networks, shortly described below. This will give the network capability to handle variable bit rate traffic, therefore allowing a different approach in the design of the correspondent codecs.

New algorithms should be designed to allow constant image quality using a variable bit-rate in the transmission according to the information content of the image sequence. This will increase the efficiency of the utilization of all resources. As a direct consequence higher quality can be achieved for the lower bit rate codecs and smaller average bit-rate is possible even when the same quality level is maintained for the high quality codecs.

VBR codecs will not be standardized before de 90's. It is believed that a good quality for business use may be achieved using average bit rates below 5Mbit/s.

Electronic archive of images requires coding for the compression of image information for storage and transmission. There is presently considerable activity at ISO in order to define standards for colour pictures and moving image sequences.

The JPEG (Joint Photographers Expert Group) of ISO/IEC and CCITT is now coming to a final decision on a recommendation for a photographic image compression technique for future image storage and communication applications, that will have strong impact on all image applications. The standard will apply to still-frame continuous tone gray-scale or colour images and will satisfy a number of predetermined conditions: ability to produce quality images at a wide range of compression rates and to provide progressive or sequential image build-up. Transmission is essentially aiming at the digital 64kbit/s channels. At present the committee is selecting one of three so far winning algorithms: ADCT (proposed by ESPRIT Project PICA), ABAC (proposed by IBM) and BSPC (proposed by Japanese Natural Image Standardization Group) [8].

In parallel with this activity a call for proposals was initiated by the MPEG (Experts Group on Moving Picture Coding), group set up under WG8 of SC2 of the joint ISO/JECT Technical Committee, in order to define a standard for Coded Representation of Motion Pictures for Digital Storage Media, having a maximum of 1.5Mbit/s, applicable in particular to magnetic and optical storage media.

Algorithms must be suitable to store moving image and sound in combination and must allow interactivity (reverse playback, random access, fast forward), compatibility with telecommunication and broadcasting, etc. The group will aim at a Draft Proposal by September 1990.

A standard like this will open entirely new perspectives in existing image services. Coding required by this applications has specific requirements but in general terms the problem is close to the VBR coding situation. Very fast developments are expected in terms of VLSI to reduce cost of terminals to unparalleled levels. Most manufacturers of all continents are involved in these activities.

3. Network Evolution

It has been decided that present public communication networks will evolve towards an Integrated Service Digital Network (ISDN). This network must be able to transport all services, including circuit switched and packet switched traffic, that put very different requirements to the network and, up to now, have used separate specific networks. In the now started first phase of the evolution towards total integration the network will only be able to transport "lower" bit-rate traffic (up to 2Mbit/s); this is called Narrowband ISDN. The available capacity will not be enough for high quality video transmission, allowing however some of the less demanding services like picture phone and videoconference. In the final phase it will however be able to carry all types of traffic, including HDTV. This final phase of the evolution will start in the late 90's; the network is called Broadband ISDN (B-ISDN).

In any case the network interface must be the same for all types of supported applications.

The analysis of the requirements put to the network by the need to carry traffic with very different characteristics made necessary the study of all possible transfer modes, in order to select those better adapted to the identified requirements [9].

STM (Synchronous Transfer Mode), presently used in the digital telephone network, will not allow an efficient use of the bandwidth, when carrying simultaneously a number of services with very different characteristics. It involves the segmentation of the transmitted bit stream into frames and these into time slots that are rigidly allocated to a specific service. A certain time slot in each successive frame is allocated to a particular call during its duration. STD is therefore channel oriented and it cannot support fast variations in traffic.

In Packet Switched Networks, using packets with information headers processed by the network nodes, it is possible to make optimum use of all available resources, however, the need to process packet header information implies delays that may not be tolerable by certain continuous bit stream services like video or even voice channels.

Considering these difficulties Asynchronous Transfer Mode (ATM) has been proposed and it has now been decided that it will be used in the B-ISDN. In this case the information is transported in cells in such a way that dynamic sharing of network transmission and switching resources between users according to their instantaneous needs is possible. The cells have reduced header information, only used to identify virtual circuits, and not to any other functions like flow control or route selection, like in packet switched networks.

There are two access rates being considered for a broadband subscriber: 150Mbit/s and 600Mbit/s. The selection will depend on the needs of the particular subscriber.

The ATM concept will have a strong impact on video coding [10,11]. Network packetization defects, in particular cell delay jitter and cell loss, will have to be considered, and will require specific countermeasures at the terminal level. ATM network is presently in its definition phase.

The evolution of private networks will have to take these facts in consideration. Up to very recently private networks would not allow a significant degree of service integration. Standard LANs were not fast enough to allow fast data services and will not allow the transport of synchronous services.

The requests put by the evolution towards a total service integration, on one side, and the need to transport fast data as well as video services, on the other side, created the need for new improved private network standards. FDDI (Fibre Distributed Data Interface) made the first step in that direction: it is an optical fibre token ring working at 100 Mbit/s, with a special protocol to enable the use of fast data transfer between stations. A second phase of this standard, FDDI-2, is now in progress [12]. It will be compatible with present standard but it will have special provisions to integrate circuit and packet switched traffic. This will be the first private network to integrate the various kinds of traffic even if not using ATM principles.

There are presently developments in areas of great significance to the evolution of private networks and work stations.

Great attention is now given to the specification and technologies of CPN (Customer Premisses Network), within the work towards the definition of the future B-ISDN, considering the needs of a domestic or a large business subscriber. Intensive activity in this area is being supported by RACE and under CEPT.

Fundamental work in optical technologies is showing the feasibility of very much higher capacity networks, allowing a even greater degree of integration. The use of coherent technologies will allow a very large number of independent channels, with new degrees of freedom to explore previously unsuspected ideas. We can easily conceive a protocol allowing network capacity sharing for synchronous high-speed traffic together with packet switched or ATM traffic, in a LAN or MAN environment [13].

The use of such high throughput networks calls for developments in the hardware to implement the corresponding interfaces: the multimedia integrated work stations required will be very demanding in terms of processing power. New fast digital processors and processing architectures, high speed interfaces and standard buses are necessary and will certainly be developed.

All these changes will have strong impact on video transmission technologies. In fact, for long distance transmission ATM concepts will allow a much more efficient use of the transmission capacities. However, in the local distribution and for high quality image it is possible that if a large transmission capacity is available at a low cost the coding is made less complex in order to reduce terminal equipment costs and allow easy post-processing of images.

It is therefore possible to imagine a scenario in which ATM type of coding and other high compression algorithms are used in the public network, particularly for long distance transmission and/or reduced quality video services, and for local transmission and high quality services, low compression synchronous codecs will be used. This has also been proposed for the distribution of TV and HDTV services, in the local network.

4. Some Issues on the Development of PACS

The video and picture transmission areas, together with related processing hardware, will see very fast changes in the near future. In the definition of future activities this fact should be taken into account, designing the applications independently of the technologies used. There are large numbers of questions to be asked concerning the quality requirements put by the medical applications as well as the importance of the artifacts generated by the compression algorithms selected.

Approved standards should be used as much as possible. The consideration of the scenarios previously described for the transmission is important because the compatibility of PACS to be developed in medical environments with the approved standards for video or picture services, is desirable, at least at the terminal level, in order to reduce costs.

Codecs can be designed using A/D and D/A interfaces of high quality, with any necessary quality degradation done by later processing stages. This will allow the use of a variable quality of the image according to the degree of movement; static or slowly moving images could therefore be transmitted with higher resolution, because there is no need to a fast transmission of changes [14].

Development work should be concentrated on the applications themselves including specific terminal equipment that may be required, using some of the advanced communications systems available. Attention should be given to the requirements in terms of image quality, database facilities, evaluation of required services and traffic generated.

While B-ISDN is not available combination of several LANs (including FDDI) and point-to-point links and switching systems should be used [15].

An interesting area deserving special attention is the specification of image and moving image archives including fast search algorithms. These should allow a fast image search, through the use of visual, other than logical, keys. Progressive coding schemes should be preferred.

5. Present and Future Activities in Related Areas at INESC

Activity in the area of Digital Video Transmission started in 1986 as part of the SIFO Project- a Project aiming at the development of a pilot Broadband Integrated Services Digital Network, using optical Fibres.

A 153.6 Mbit/s Composite Video Codec was first developed as a means to test other SIFO subsystems, at a stage when the MUX/DEMUX generating the 153.6 Mbit/s frame were not ready. The composite video signal (PAL) is sampled at a sampling rate of 13.568 MHz with 8 bit/sample and coded in linear PCM. The digital video data is multiplexed with a digital audio channel (2048 Kbit/s), with the 153.6 Mbit/s frame synchronization word, with 139.264 Mbit/s frame synchronization word and with the empty slot signal. It is important to note that the digital video data and the associated digital audio data are formatted as a 139.264 Mbit/s frame inside the 153.6 Mbit/s frame. A fast FIFO working as an elastic buffer is used to accommodate the difference between the video data production rate (13.568 MHz) and the multiplexing rate (19.2 MHz). A sequential controller determines the timing for the insertion of the different signals. The last operation is the parallel-to-serial conversion made with a 10KH ECL device.

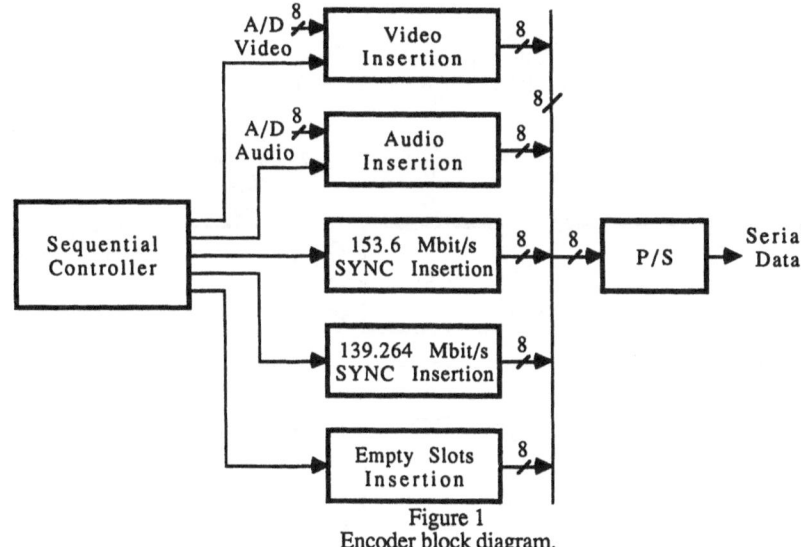

Figure 1
Encoder block diagram.

In the decoder the complementary operations are performed. A sequential controller is also used in this unit.

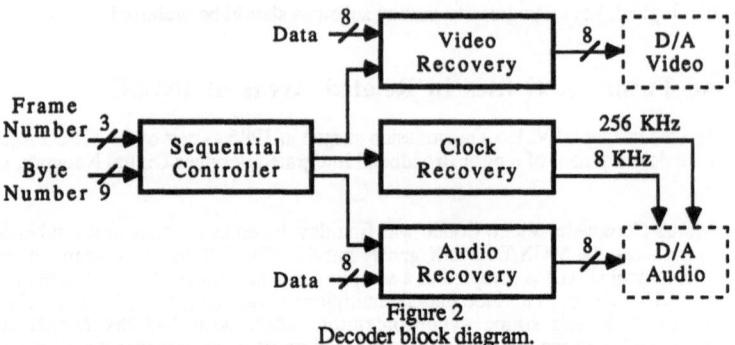

Figure 2
Decoder block diagram.

This development was completed and tested with success in June 1988, and it was demonstrated during the Preliminary Demonstration of the SIFO Project, during July 1988. The quality obtained was very good.

The main limitation of this Codec came from the fact that it requires synchronism between the sampling clock, that must be locked to the colour carrier frequency, and the network clock.

A 139.264 Mbit/s Components Video Codec was designed for the final distribution of digital video in the SIFO network. It allows the transmission of a three-component video signal and the associated stereo audio channel at a 139.264 Mbit/s rate (H4 channel).

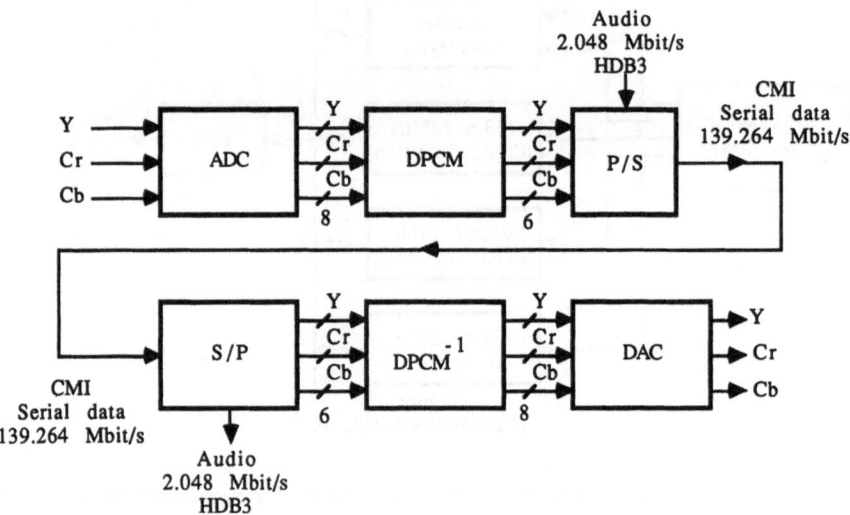

Figure 3
139.264 Mbit/s Codec block diagram.

The ADC and DAC interfaces follow the CCIR's Rec. 601. The luminance signal (Y) is sampled at a 13.5 MHz rate and the colour difference signals (Cr, Cb) are sampled at 6.75 MHz rate (Level 4:2:2).

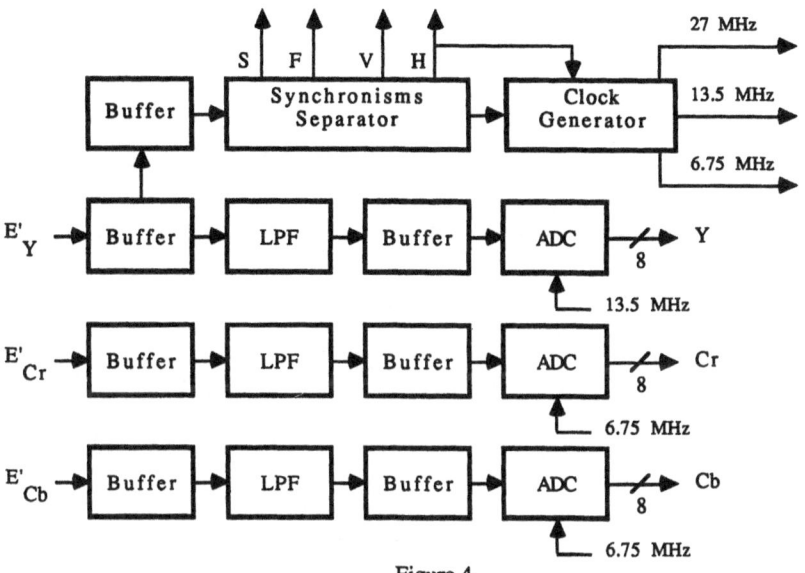

Figure 4
ADC block diagram.

Figure 5
DAC block diagram.

The bit rate obtained is 216 Mbit/s and it must compressed in order to obtain the desired transmission rate (139.264 Mbit/s). This is accomplished using the hybrid DPCM coding method proposed by Van Bull, converting 8-bit PCM words into 6-bit DPCM words and eliminating the video signal horizontal blanking period. The prediction is made using the previous sample.

As the data rate produced is different from the transmission rate, it is necessary to accommodate the difference between them. This is accomplished with a stuffing scheme implemented with elastic buffers.

The audio is received in a 2.048 Mbit/s frame and is formatted with the video data for transmission. The frame used is a 139.264 Mbit/s similar to one of the frames recommended for multiplexing purposes in the Rec. G.700 series. CMI code is used for transmission.

In parallel with this activity in the area of standard TV transmission, a 2 Mbit/s Video Codec was designed to provide transmission of monochrome video pictures over 2048 Kbit/s digital channels, with a picture quality sufficient for surveillance purposes. It accepts one standard monochrome or colour (PAL) video signal with 625 lines and 50 field/s. Processing is reduced in order to keep the costs reduced and development time short.

The signal is bandlimited to 2 MHz and sampled at a frequency of 5 MHz, locked to the video wave-form, producing 320 samples per complete line. Only 256 samples per active line are transmitted. The signal is coded with uniformly quantized PCM with 6 bit per sample.

In order to transmit this video signal in a 2048 Kbit/s channel the signal must be further compressed. To achieve this the video blanking periods are not transmitted (but the information of their temporal location is kept for future insertion of timing reference codes) and the digitized video signal is vertically and temporally subsampled and coded in DPCM with 3 bit per sample. As a result, only 286 lines per frame (or 143 lines per field) and only 8 frames per second (or 16 fields per second) are transmitted.

After these operations the video data is applied to a buffer memory whose function is to smooth the irregular data rate and adapt it to the constant bit rate of the 2.048 Mbit/s stream. In this buffer memory the video data is expanded along the time of the suppressed lines, frames and video blanking signals.

Timing reference codes must be inserted at this point to insure the proper recovery at the receiving end of the video signal format. They consist of a sequence of three 6-bit words, being the two first ones a fixed identification preamble with PCM forbidden values and the third one containing information about video synchronization and odd/even field identification.

The data stream is then formatted in a frame according to the CCITT G.700 Recommendations.

This Codec is now fully completed and tested.

In the area of picture archiving systems interfaces were designed for the acquisition and display of two-tone pictures in an Optical Disk Archive System. Facsimile standards were adopted for acquisition and display. Compression/Decompression algorithms are implemented in the display controller in order to allow the use of more efficient algorithms and the transmission of the compressed files.

Ongoing and Future Activities:

Work will soon start on a 34 Mbit/s Video Codec, with quality appropriate for video distribution. The processing will follow ITU available Recommendations. For the processing particular attention will be given to the DCT (Discrete Cosine Transform).

The development of a VBR Codec and participation in the development of a px64kbit/s are also in preparation.

In order to integrate all possible coding activities in a common hardware a flexible architecture codec is now being conceived.

The design of an integrated multimedia work station (ESTIMULO), based on Multibus II and a UNIX like operating system, and including several standard interfaces (FDDI, Token Ring, Ethernet, ISDN) and special graphic and image handling facilities is in progress.

The Optical Disk Archive system is being upgraded to efficiently store and display colour and gray scale black and white pictures. This development will follow the standardization activities in the area.

Experiments will continue with the 2 Mbit/s Surveillance Codec developed, aiming at transmission in LANs, using conditional replenishment techniques.

On the network side, we stress our involvement in advanced network development, through the participation in European projects (ex. RACE ATD and BCPN, ESPRIT II UCOL).

6. References:

[1] Report 1089 CCIR, 1986
[2] H. Murakami, H. Hashimoto, Y. Hatori "Quality of Band-Compressed TV Services", IEEE Communications Magazine, Oct. 1988
[3] H. G. Musmann, P. Pirsch, H.J.Gallert "Advances in Picture Coding", Proceedings IEEE, vol. 73, n⁰4, April 1985
[4] F. Kretz, D. Nasse "Digital Television and Coding" Proceedings of IEEE, vol. 73,m n⁰4, April 1985
[5] R. J. Clark "Transform Coding of Images", Academic Press, 1985   (ISBN 0-12-175730-7)
[6] A. N. Netravali, J. O. Limb "Picture Coding: a Review" Proceedings of IEEE, vol.68,n⁰3, March 1980
[7] A. Jain "Image Data Compression: a Review", Proceedings of IEEE, vol.69, n⁰3, March 1981
[8] G. P. Hudson, H. Yasuda "The Selection of a Still Picture Compression Technique for International Standardization", PCS, Torino, Italy, Sept. 1988
[9] P. Gonet, P. Adam, J. P. Coudreuse "Asynchronous Time-Division Switching: The Way to Flexible Broadband Communication Networks" Seminar, Zurich, 1986
[10] G. Karlsson, M. Vetterli "Subband Coding of Video for Packet   Networks", Optical Engineering, vol. 27, n⁰7, July 1988
[11] W. Verbiest, L. Pinnoo, B. Voeten "Impact of ATM Concept on   Video Coding", IEEE SAC, vol. SAC-6, n⁰9, Dec. 1988
[12] F. E. Ross "FDDI - a Tutorial", IEEE Com. Magazine, vol. 24, n⁰5, May 1986
[13] A. Fioretti, S. Forcesi "UCOL: a Concept for an Ultra-Wideband Coherent Optical Man", OCTIMA International Workshop, Rome, January 1989
[14] L. Chiariglioni, S. Fontolan, M. Guglielmo, F. Tommasi "A   Variable Resolution Video Codec for Low Bit-Rate   Applications", IEEE SAC, vol. SAC-5, n⁰7, August 1987
[15] R. Castanet "High Speed LAN for Image Transmission", EFOC/LAN 87, Basel, Switzerland, June 1987

Medical Work Stations for Computer Assisted Radiology

Heinz U. Lemke

Tecnical University of Berlin . Franklinstrasse 28-29 D-1000 Berlin 10 F.R.G.

1 Introduction

Computer Assisted Radiology (CAR) is the application of computer and communication technology in radiological and related medical activities for the generation, processing, management and communication of medical images. Its principle aim is to improve the qualitative impression, the quantitative measurement and the communication of medical images, relating to the state of health of a patient.

With these characteristics, CAR represents a natural progression in the medical usage of tools and techniques from early history of medicine to our present day. Occasionally, however, quantum steps are being taken during the evolution of tools for medical purposes, such as the discovery of X-rays by C. Röntgen in 1895 or the employment of the computer for tomographic image reconstruction by G. Hounsfield in 1972. Both have introduced a new line of tools for medical diagnosis and therapy planning. Each event was formally recognised by awarding the Nobel prize.

Although computers have been employed in medical imaging for some time, such as, for example, very specialised gamma camera displays in nuclear medicine, G. Hounsfield with computer tomography, and later others with magnetic resonance imaging, computed radiography, etc. have set the basis of CAR.

Digital imaging is the prerequisit for CAR. Employment of CAR methods are, therefore, dependent on the acceptance and usage of digital imaging for medical diagnosis and therapy planning. At present, digital imaging occupies between 20 to 30 percent of imaging procedures in modern hospitals. Dependent on this, CAR still remains a tool for specific purposes. Predictions are made, however, that by the early 1990's, 50 percent of all medical imaging procedures will be digital in origin (cf. Ref. 1). Estimates on the growth of the most important digital imaging procedures between 1985 and 1995 are shown in Table 1-1 (cf. Ref. 2). With a parallel development of computer and communication technology being adapted to medical imaging requirements, CAR is expected, by the turn of the millennium, to be seen as a general tool for medical diagnosis and therapy planning. Various subspecialities in the computer and communication disciplines are contributing towards this, see chapters III and IV. The basis for this, however, is an understanding and subsequent augmentation of the activities within the field of radiology.

2 Radiology

2.1 Diagnostic Pathway

Radiology fulfills the commonly accepted definition of a discipline, as defined by a system of

a) objects and definitions, i.e. medical images of patients and the definitions of image parts,
b) relationships, i.e. of parts within images and between images,
c) body of propositions and hypotheses, i.e. meaning of particular instantiations of images and their parts,
d) methods and techniques for image generation, modelling, analysis,verification and description, i.e. consultation and reporting on patient specific imaging procedures.

Components a) to c) are the basis for d) which in turn may be referred to as the diagnostic pathway. Fig. 2-1 shows an activity flowchart of the diagnostic pathway. Medical imaging, interpreting, consulting and reporting represent the heart of the radiological activity.

Different types of medical and support personnel may be contributing towards the activities in the pathway, as indicated in Fig. 2-2. Some of these have direct contact with the patient, others spend more time on producing and handling the patient-specific medical records. Because the medical record occupies a central position in most health care environments, its form and access facilities are of critical importance.

2.2 Medical Record

In the process of medical diagnosis and therapy, information on a patient is usually presented by means of the written word, pictures, graphics and the spoken word. For a particular patient, the sum-total of this information may be labelled the medical record (MR).

Typically, a MR is recorded on charts, films, computer storage and, most important, in the mind of the medical care team. Different types of paper charts and other non-computerised varieties of patient data carriers make tracing of MR's difficult. Paper charts, for example, exhibit several deficiencies (Ref. 3) :

- Illegibility. A variable portion of the medical record cannot be accurately deciphered because of scribbled notation.
- Incompleteness. The record lacks certain facts that are necessary for proper interpretation of the care given to a specific patient.
- Ambiguity. There exists a lack of precision in the definition of diagnosis, treatment, and follow-up instructions
- Disorganisation. The specific logical portions of the medical record are not defined clearly, making later review of a specific portion both time-consuming and difficult.
- Inaccuracy. "Mistakes" in dictation and notation have not been resolved.
- Poor Coding. The specific "codes" used for reporting purposes do not accurately represent the "true" conditions, treatments, or follow- up status of the patient.
- Tardiness. There are delays in the completion and processing of the medical record.

Problems which may be caused by these deficiencies (Ref. 3):
- Frustration for patients, doctors, nurses, and other users of the record.
- Inefficiency in the provision of care.
- Diagnosis and treatment errors.
- Poor quality communication with other members of the health care system.
- Billing problems.
- Poor medical-legal defence.
- Audit difficulties.
- Low morale.

In the interest of a patient-oriented health care system, there are a number of important, if not vital, requirements on how the information in the MR should be organised and used, e.g. there should be (Ref. 4):
a) reliable linkage of all patient-specific information into one MR (sometimes referred to as a multi-media MR),
b) access to the information in the MR at the right place, in the right time, for the right people, and
c) flexible conferencing and consulting mode facilities, using MRs and all modes of communication (i.e; word, picture and voice communication).

In addition, there are some desirable features of data representation and processing for the medical practitioner, e. g. there should be:
d) uniform, structured and easy to understant data representation of MRs,
e) easily extendable MRs,
f) safe, protected and easily accessible MRs,
g) speedy processing facilities on MRs.

Using appropriate computer and communication systems, CAR is a tool with the potential to satisfy the above requirements.

2.3   Computer Assisted Radiology

Computer assistance may be realised at various positions in the pathway of Fig. 2.1, as indicated in Fig. 2-3. This is usually achieved with specialized medical workstations which form part of, or have access to, a computer and/or communication network.

Overall support for clerical and administrative activities can be provided within the radiological department by a radiological information system (RIS). Communication to the outside of the radiological departement is realised via interface from RIS to a hospital information system (HIS).

Image processing can be applied to image formation and reconstruction. Image handling and communication is supported by medical workstations integrated into a picture archiving and communication system (PACS). A PACS may be part of a local area network (LAN) connected to a wide area network (WAN) which could then allow teleradiological services.

A large number of image display and manipulation facilities supporting the activities of the diagnostic pathway may also be realized with medical workstations. Integrated into appropriate communication networks, they provide the potential for radiology to occupy an increasingly important position for servicing other medical disciplines, such as orthopaedics, radiology, neurology, radiotherapy as well as general and specialized surgery.

3   Computers in Radiology

3.1   Medical Workstations

Many of the requirements resulting from the production, processing, management and communication of MRs can be satisfied by using medical workstations (MWSs) in communication networks. A number of such MWSs with different user functions have been developed, and are being used in various clinical settings.

3.1.1   User Requirements

The attributes of the image and non-image data determine the type of functions the MWS should support. S. Hori (cf. Ref. 5) has pointed out a number of data qualities which should be considered for medical imaging workstations:

- Printing characteristics - for CRT displays, the character size and font for text and for images, the matrix size and bit depth.
- Timing - the rate and duration of data presentation. This is under almost absolute control of the radiologist reading films. For data presented on CRTs, however, this may not be the case.
- Order - the position of data relative to other data.
- Grouping - the tendency of some data elements to have cohesion to other data elements, e.g. to satisfy anatomic or time relationships.
- Formatting - the physical arrangement of the data so as to impart meaning. Radiologist film "sorting" behaviour is very likely to be involved in this aspect of data quality.
- Scaling - dimensioning the data to a particular standard. For imaging, this would refer to altering the physical size of some data displays to match others.
- Transiency - the transformation of data from one form into another during use or communication. Interpretation of images is one major example and forming images from parametric data is another.
- Quantity - the amount of data present. Radiologist focus on a smaller group of images (if multiple), effectively limiting the data quantity.
- Complexity - the variety of functions implicit or explicit in the data. Medical image data tends to be very complex, especially if multidimensional .
- Relevancy - refers to how noisy the data is. For medical imaging, there is a large component of structure noise present; whether data is noise or signal, is task dependent (Ref. 5).

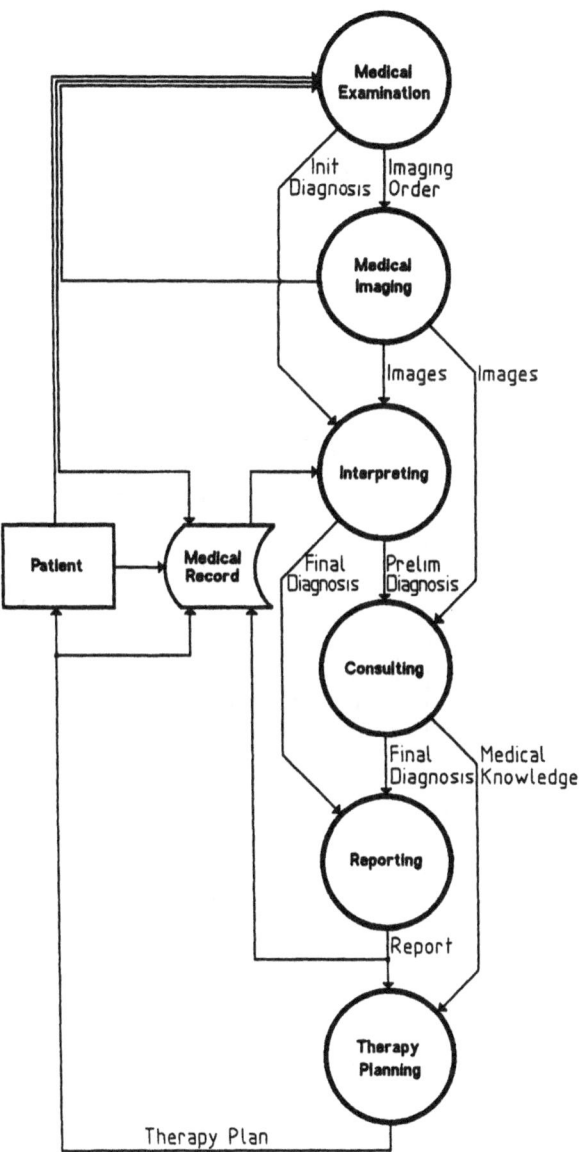

Fig 2-1 Activities in Diagnostic Pathway

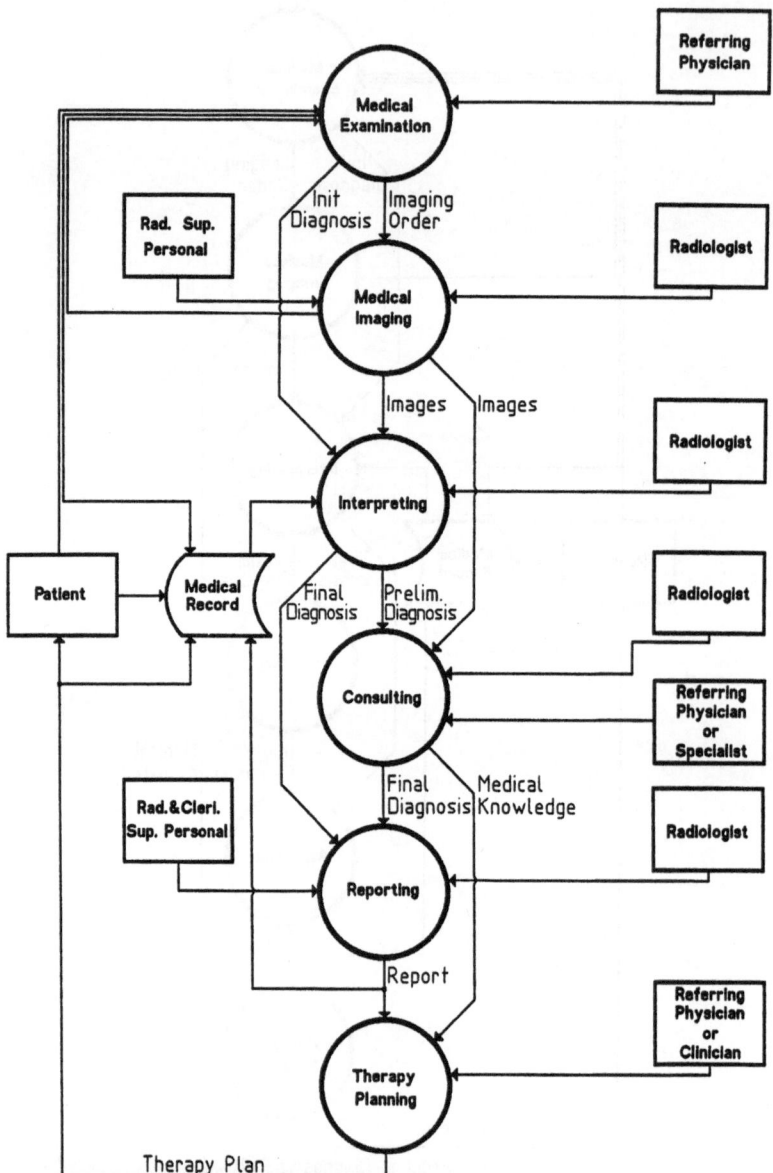

Fig. 2-2 Personnel in Diagnostic Pathway

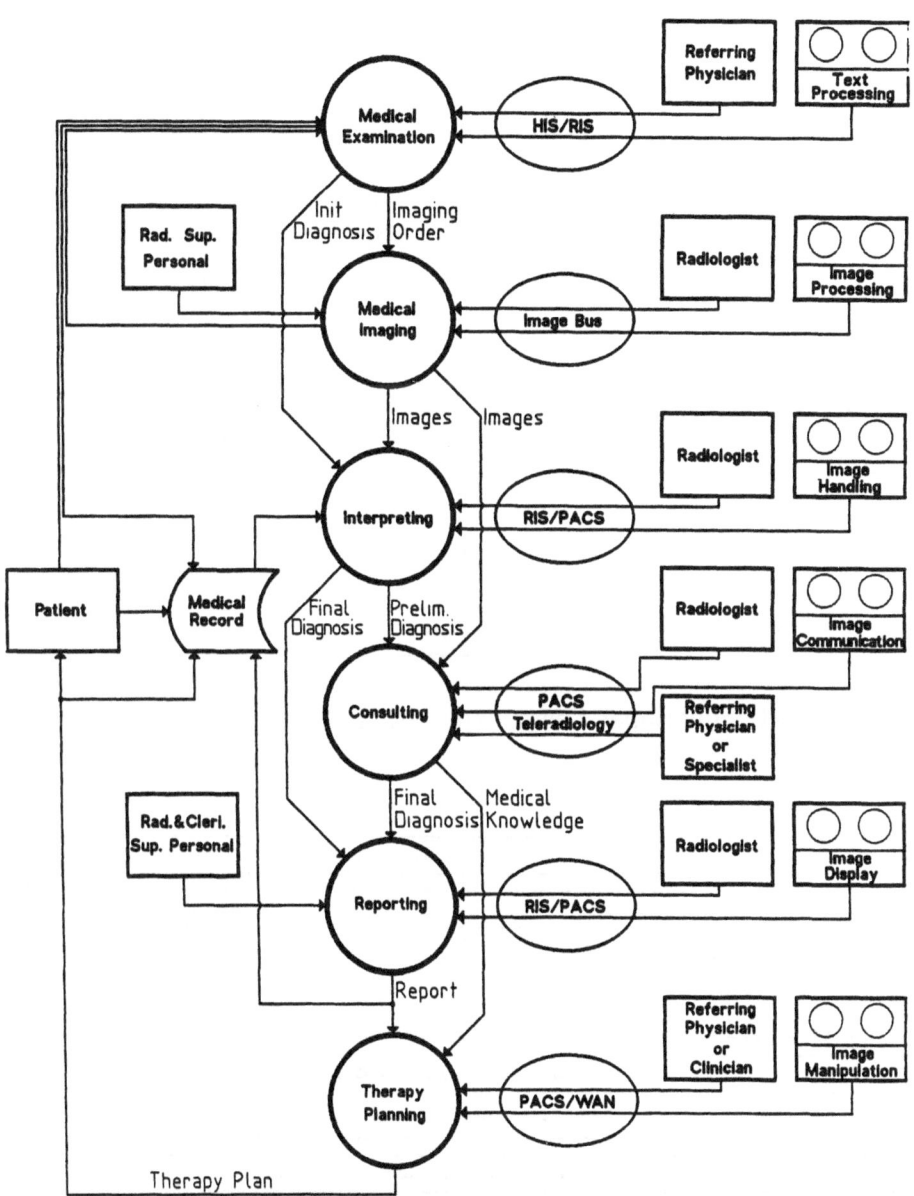

Fig. 2-3 Computer and Communication Systems in Diagnostic Pathway

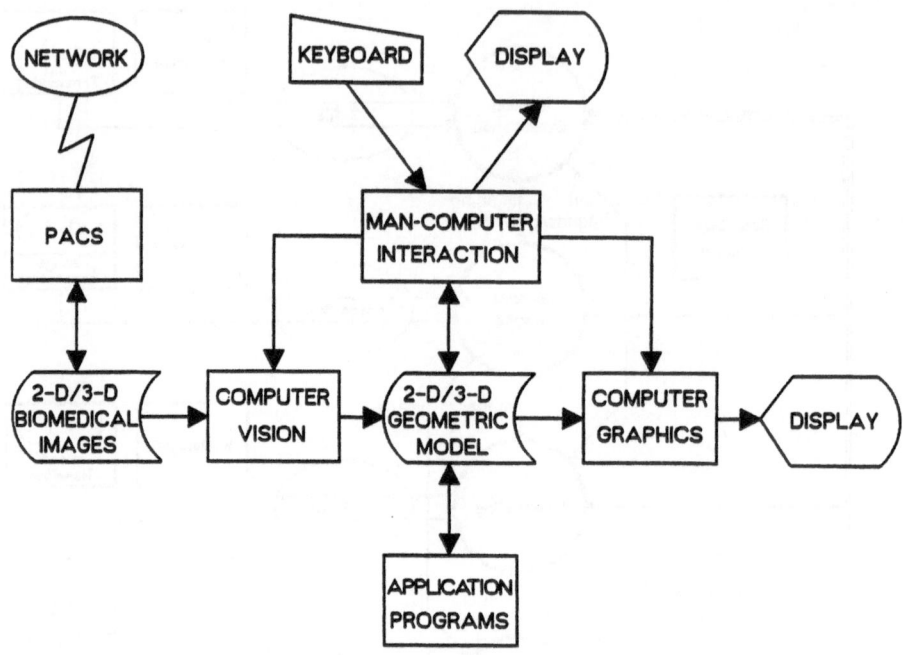

Fig. 3-1 Functional Components of a Medical Workstation

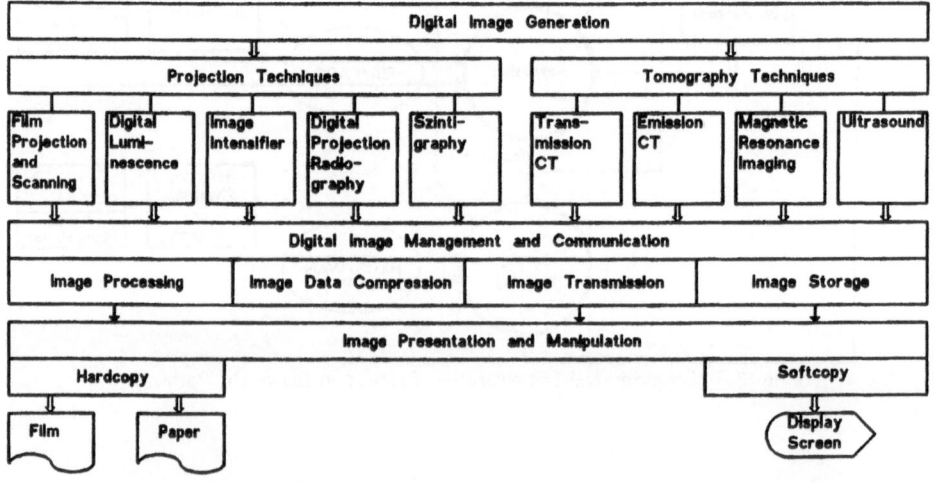

Fig. 3-2 Digital Image Generation and Presentation

The information processing functions for medical image data are derived from techniques of subspeciality areas of computer science, such as computer vision, computer graphics, modelling and man-computer-interaction, see Fig. 3-1. A summary of possible functions for viewing, reporting and high capability visualisation and manipulation stations is given in Appendix A 1, (S. Pizer, personal communication).

3.1.2   Computer Vision

Computer vision algorithms may be applied to the preprocessing, segmentation and analysis of images. They should take account of the psychovisual behaviour of the human observer, and should provide quantitative information on processed images.

A very important emerging aspect is the a priori knowledge representation and model driven analysis of images. With this, concepts of machine intelligence are increasingly being employed in computer vision.

3.1.3   Computer Graphics

The most important computer graphics techniques available for 2-dimensional and/or 3-dimensional display are:

a)   rotational, transational and scaling transformations,
b)   parallel and perspective projections,
c)   kinetic depths cues,
d)   stereoscopic viewing,
e)   hidden line and hidden surface removal,
f)   illumination models, and
g)   dynamic voxel representations.

Modelling is often taken to be part of computer graphics and is concerned with the computer representation of geometry. Current techniques evolve around polygones, cuberilles, B-splines and cubic splines representations. For composite medical imaging, combined modelling with the above and other techniques, will become increasingly important. Extraction of 2-dimensional and 3-dimensional metric informatin must be possible, particularly for diagnostic purposes. Model shaping operations should be provided for therapeutic and teaching types of medical workstations.

3.1.4   Man-Computer-interaction

User-friendly man-computer-interaction implies appropriate interface design for the handling of alphanumeric, picture, graphic, voice and tactile information. As yet, there are not generally accepted "human engineering" concepts on how to design this interface. Current man-computer-interaction systems for medical imaging are ad hoc designs. A number of ergonomic factors have been suggested by S.C. Horii (cf. Ref. 5), G.v. Voigt (cf. Ref. 8) an others, for example:

1.   Minimum dependency on keyboards
2.   Few steps for often used functions and macro facilities
3.   Robust
4.   Undo functions
5.   Predefined window width and window level for imaging
6.   Work surface (incl. light boxes)
7.   Small distance between monitors
8.   Tilt/swift monitor mounts
9.   Most used controls in comfortable positions
10.   Convenient seating, handedness and display partitioning
11.   Simple procedural access
12.   Organ and/or image oriented information coding of form, time and colour
13.   User selectable audible input cues
14.   Systems busy indicator
15.   Spill proof
16.   Appropriate real time response

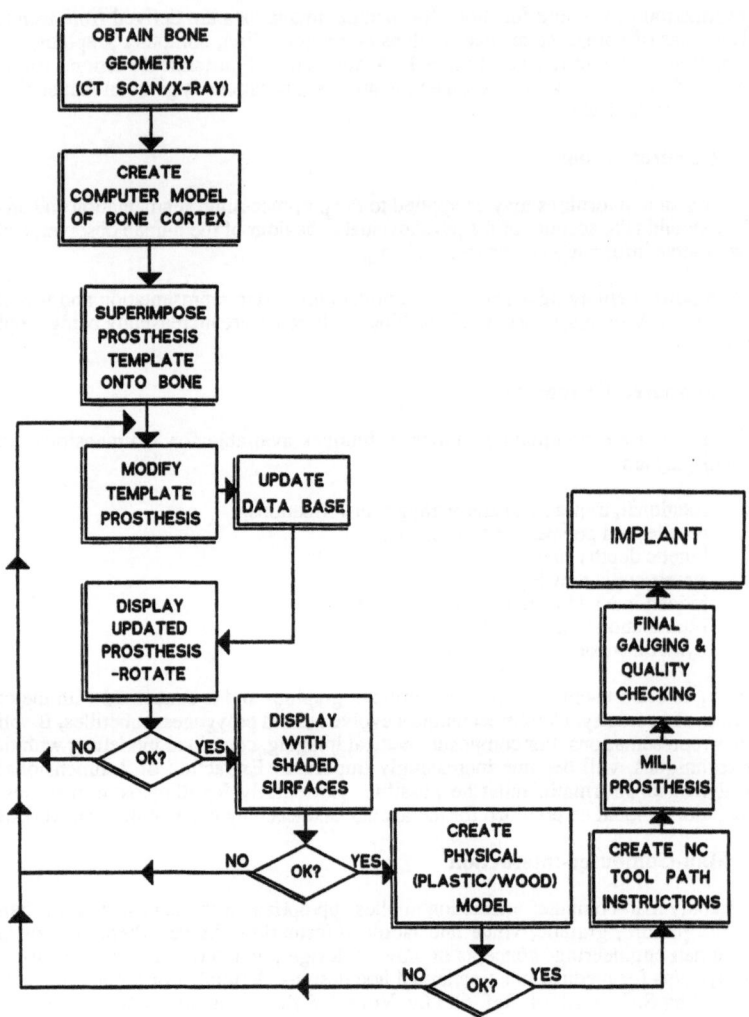

Fig.3-3 Flowchart of Design Process for Patient-specific Prothesis

17. Appropriate sound and light levels
18. Aesthetics
19. Convenient physical access
20. Hard copy facility

A very important issue still to be resolved is to ensure compatibility of MWS functions. The aim should be to allow for upward functional compatibility, e.g. from 2-D diagnostic workstations to 4-D teaching workstations.

3.2 Computer Assistance in Diagnostic Pathway

3.2.1   Medical Examination

Apart from making patient data available (perhaps retrieved from a file and presented on a display terminal) little computer assistance can be (should be) employed at this activity. The medical exam activity is usually being carried out by a clinician or referring physician and, except in emergencies, relatively seldom by a radiologist. Result documentation and further test scheduling may be supported by a HIS and/or RIS.

3.2.2   Diagnostic Imaging

In addition to X-rays, many different physical principles may be employed in the scanning of a patient. Further examples are magnetic resonance and ultrasound as well as photon and positron emission in nuclear medicine. Computer assisted medical imaging is the process by which the signals of the scanning procedures are digitised and processed by the computer to generate an image.

Further processing and management of these images are possible (e.g. filtering, enhancement etc.) before presentation either as hard or soft copy, see Fig. 3-2.

Each patient imaging procedure requires, depending on imaging modality and suspected pathology, a characteristic set of images with an exected spatial, temporal and contrast resolution. The data volume per image for a particular modality may range from a few kilobytes in nuclear medicine to several megabytes in digital radiography, see Table 3-1.

3.2.3   Image Interpretaion

After processing, the medical images are reviewed and interpreted by the medical specialist. Additional medical data, such as the initial diagnosis of the referring physician and/or patient history and previous medical images, may be consulted in this process.

Computer assistance can be applied here by using appropriate medical image workstations with functions simulating or surpassing the features of light boxes and alternators. A multitude of image data handling functions has been developed for these types of diagnostic medical workstations.

3.2.4   Consulting and Reporting

In the consulting and reporting steps, a diagnosis is finalised and appropriately reported. Generation and distribution of the report represent the main service function of the radiological department. The quality of this service is measured on accuracy, comprehensibility and timeliness of the report.

To improve accuracy, a consultation process may be initiated allowing access to further medical knowledge. Such consultation may be realized through cooperation with a medical colleague or through access to a data bank and/or expert system. Furthermore, actual writing of the report can be carried out by support staff or by automated systems which may include speech recognition functions.

Comprehensibility of the report can be achieved through effective use of image augmenting features. They should be adjusted to the needs of the recipient of the report. Typical functions for example, for projection images are: region of interest enhancements, markers, labelling, scaling, shifting, etc.. In addition, series of tomographic images may reconstructed to provide coronal, sagittal, paraxial, curved or 3-D voxel and surface displays. For some medical specialities, such as neurology, cardiology, orthopaedics and ENT, images are very important in the diagnostic process. They often profit from additional 3-D qualitative and quantitative data, see Table 3-2. Radiological support staff may here be employed to provide these imaging features.

Timeliness of the report is related to the needed availability of diagnostic information for therapy. It may refer to time critical procedures, such as in trauma, or to relatively time independent events, such as in imaging for reconstructive surgery.

3.2.5   Therapy Planning

Many sectional image sequences are difficult to interpret anatomically. Computer graphics methods for 3-D reconstruction, modelling and manipulation can improve this situation and assist in therapy and teaching efforts.

Although not generally part of radiology (with the occasional exception of radiation therapy), therapy planning may be assisted by computing facilities in the radiological department. Basically, it consists of providing the desired patient image and modelling data which can then be further manipulated within the respective medical discipline, see Table 3-3. Possible examples are the application of computer graphics to custom-designed implants in orthopaedics, and modelling and display of anatomy for surgery.

Fig. 3-3 shows a flowchart of the design process for patient-specific prothesis (cf. Ref. 6). Techniques from computer aided design and manufacturing are usually incorporated in the computer modelling, displays and manipulation.

In general, surface and volumetric computer graphic rendering methods can be applied, see Fig. 3-4 and 3-5 respectively. In some cases, stereoviewing appears to be useful, see Fig. 3-6.

How much of these services will be provided by radiology in a typical clinical setting is still unclear.

4   Communication in Radiology

4.1   Communication Systems

Implicit in Fig. 2-3 are a number of communication paths for the transfer of information. Critical for an effective health care system is, in particular, inter-human communication. It may be carried out between referring physician and patient, radiologist and supporting staff, radiologist and medical specialists or radiologist and referring physician and clinician. Traditionally, these communication paths are established by the spoken word, written documents or visits.

With digital imaging, computer assisted methods for image management, and modern digital communication technology, new types of communication channels are being realised. They augment the traditional human communication paths or allow for new types of human-computer interaction. Various health care zones and associated users may be part of a distributed information management and communication system, see Fig. 4-1 (Ref. 7). They may be served by different types of communication networks.

Several concepts and realizations of picture archiving and communication systems and teleradiology systems demonstrate this point. There exist open and closed systems, single-vendor and multi-vendor systems, star, bus, and ring topologies, as well as a multitude of different types of terminals which may start from simple, up to highly sophisitcated workstations and optical archiving systems.

First generation PAC systems, usually closed systems based on slow ($\leq$ 10-50 Mbit/sec.) LANs, have been realized in zone 1 of Fig. 4.1. Gradually, second generation open systems, based

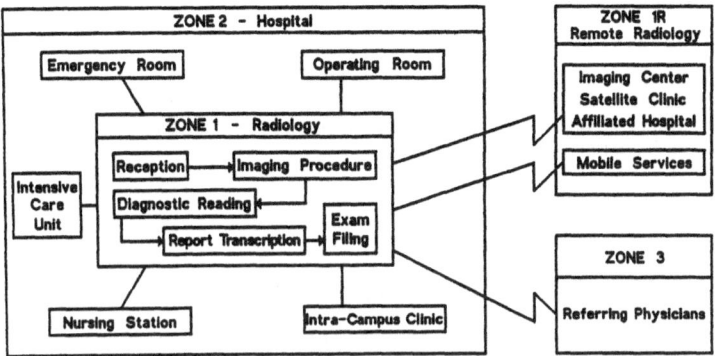

Fig 4 1 Operational Zone Model of the Radiological Community

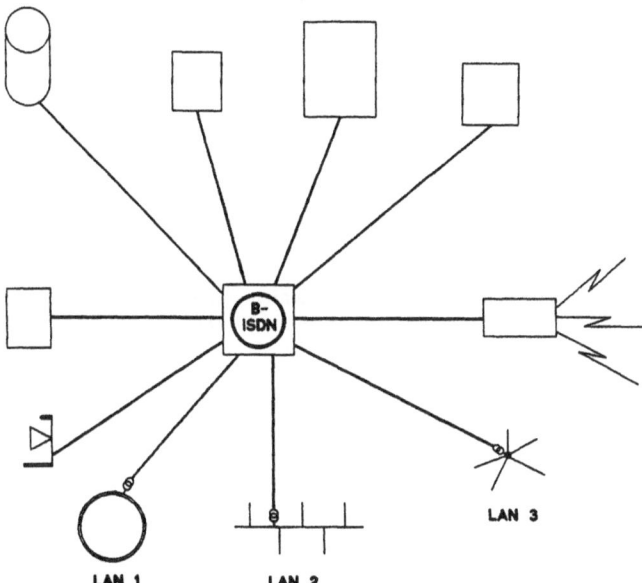

Fig. 4-2 Network Topology for Centralised High Capacity Transmission

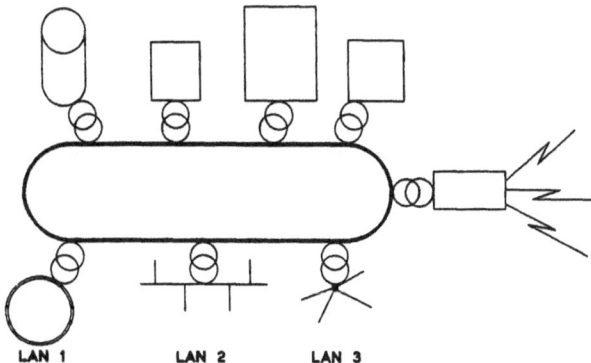

Fig. 4-3 Network Topology for Distributed High Capacity Transmission

on faster (>50 Mibt/sec.) and standardised image communication LANs, are evolving. They may also serve zone 2.

A characteristic of image transmission networks is, that they should be high-speed. Furthermore, to allow for network growth and long life they should be open systems, oriented along international standards. In addition, they should be distributed and allow broadband communication, for example to zone 1R and 3.

4.2 Communication in Diagnostic Pathway

4.2.1 Medical Examination and Imaging Scheduling

Initial creation of the MR and communication of its content to various locations may be provided by HIS and/or RIS functions. The HIS provides administrative functions supporting entry and management of patient demographic data, order entry, exam scheduling and status data, reporting, billing, etc. RIS includes some HIS-functions, but, in addition, some specific radiological functions, such as film library management, interpretation, transcription and radiological reporting are also available. Both HIS or RIS are typically realized on traditional hospital and department-wide communication networks for text transmission.

4.2.2 Medical Imaging

Communication within the digital imaging system and local processing systems require high bandwidth image transfer channels. Specialized parallel bus-systems with up to 100 megabits per second transfer rate may be required for real-time display of large volumes of image data, as for example in digital angiography or other dynamic medical imaging procedures.

4.2.3 Interpretation

Interpretation may be supported by PACS, which provides short, medium and long term storage along with various hard and soft copy display facilities. Certain functions are shared with RIS. Some interface problems between RIS and PACS still remain to be solved.

For interpretation, it is necessary to have fast access to new and old images from various imaging modalities held in a patient file. This demands high speed local area networks with an open network architecture to allow for the integration of imaging devices and other system components from multiple vendors.

4.2.4 Consulting and Reporting

Local consulting may be supported by PACS. Long distance consulting requires some kind of teleradiology system using wide area network facilities. Teleradiology facilities are being developed in many countries using smallband and broadband ISDN or similar network infrastructures. Possible topologies for such networks are shown in Fig. 4-2 for centralised and in Fig. 4-3 for distributed transmission (cf. Ref. 2). The reporting function may be supported by RIS and PACS facilities.

4.2.5 Therapy Planning

Preparatory work for therapy planning may be carried out on the local facility. For certain specialized tasks it is feasible that specialised health care centres can provide this service. The usually required long distance access may be realized via wide area networks. Again, the network facilities indicated in Fig. 4-2 and 4-3 are useful for this purpose.

5 Impact of Computer Assisted Radiology

Qualitative and quantitative handling of medical images using modern information technology is advancing in an evolutionary manner. Communication of medical images, however, may be realized

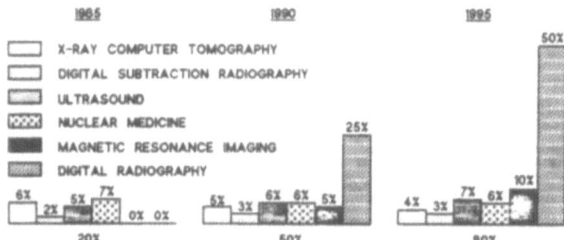

	1985	1990	1995

□ X-RAY COMPUTER TOMOGRAPHY
□ DIGITAL SUBTRACTION RADIOGRAPHY
▨ ULTRASOUND
▨ NUCLEAR MEDICINE
■ MAGNETIC RESONANCE IMAGING
▨ DIGITAL RADIOGRAPHY

Table 1-1 Estimates of Digital Imaging Procedures in a University Hospital

Digital Imaging Modality	Spatial Res.	Contrast Res. Bits/Pixel	Data Volume Mbyte/Image
Dig. Radiography	2048 x 2048	12 bits	6.00
Dig. Subtr. Ang.	1024 x 1024	12 bits	1.50
X-Ray CT	512 x 512	12 bits	0.40
Nuclear Mag. Res.	512 x 512	16 bits	0.50
Nuclear Medicine	256 x 256	8 bits	0.07
Ultrasound	512 x 512	8 bits	0.25

Table 3-1 Data Volumes for Digital Imaging Modalities

Diagnosis / Med. Speciality	Morphology		Function	
	Qualitative	Quantitative	Qualitative	Quantitative
Neurology	Position and extent of lesion	Surface areas and volumes	Diffusion of metabolic markers	Composit imaging data
Cardiology	Shape of cardiovascular structures	Flow velocities and volumes	Extent of normal vs deficient circulat.	Time tracking of markers
Othopaedics	Position and degree of deformations	Bone density and dimensional data	Degrees of freedom	Stress analysis
Ent	Position and extent of lesion	Distances between obj. of interest	- - -	- - -

Table 3-2 Qualitative and Quantitative Diagnostic Imaging Features

Therapy / Med. Speciality	Surgery	Radiation
Neurology	Target point finding and path simulation	Isodose distribution
Cardiology	Shape and metrics of transplantation objects	- - -
Othopaedics	Custom design of endoprothetic devices	- - -
Ent	Collision detection	Isodose distribution

Table 3-3 Image and Modelling Features for Surgery and Radiation Therapy

through entirely new concepts in health care communication infrastructures. This can only be achieved through a new way of thinking by patient, radiologist, physician , engineer, administrator, legislator and ever politician. Each group of people involved , however, has established many different perceptions and patterns of thinking when confronting issues relating to computer and communication technology in medicine.

These perceptions often reflect the divergence of human activity towards technical progress on one hand and the understanding of social and ethical implications on the other. The perceptions of a particular group on the advantages and shortcomings of modern tools and systems in medicine will determine the group's cooperation towards their realisation. Development of CAR systems should therefore be accompanied by investigations into their social implications.

References

1) Lodwick G.S. and Taaffe J.L.: "Radiology Systems of the Nineties: Meeting the Challenge of Change." *Journal of Digital Imaging*, 1988; 1, n°.1, pp 4 -12.

2) Lemke H.U. : "Picture Archiving and Communication Systems." Proceedings of the 5th International Symposium on the Planning of Radiological Departments - ISPRAD V, Editors : Chiesa, A, Gasparotti, R., Maroldi, R., Florence, Italy. April 1988, pp 198-208.

3) Kuslich S.D. and Cynthia M.P. : "The Human Element in the Design of Computer Assisted Orthopedic Inpatient Medical Record Systems." Use of Computers in Orthopaedics, Editors : Kuslich, S.D., Vannier, M.W. and Marsh, J.L..*The Orthopedic Clinics of North America*. Oct. 1986; 17, n°.4, pp 527-539.

4) Lemke H.U., Stiehl H.S., Scharnweber H., Jackel D.: "Applications of Picture Processing, Image Analysis and Computer Graphic Techniques to Cranial CT scans." Proceedings of Conference on Computer Aided Analysis of Radiological Images, IEEE, Newport Beach, California, USA. June 1979, pp 341-354.

5) Horii S.C.: "An Eclectic Look at a Viewing Station Design." Proceedings of Medical Imaging II, Editors: Schneider, R.H. and Dwyer III, S.J..*SPIE* Newport Beach, California, Febr. 1988; 914, part B, pp 920-928.

6) Bechthold J.E.: "Application of Computer Graphics in the Design of Custom Orthopedic Implant." Use of Computer in Orthopaedics, Ed: Kuslich, S.D., Vannier, M.W. and Marsh, J.L., *The Orthopedic Clinics of North America*. Oct 1986;17, n° 4, pp 605-612.

7) Ricca S.P., Huynh T.C. and Kong N.: "Impact of Advanced Fibre Optics and ISDN Technologies on PACS Networking ." Proceedings of Medical Imaging III, Editors: Schneider, R.H., Dwyer III, S;J. and Jost, R.G., *SPIE*, Newport Beach, California. Febr. 1989; 1093.

8) v. Voigt G.: "Betrachtung der Mensch-Computer-Interaktion eines bilddatenorientierten medizinischen Arbeitsplatzes für computergestützte Diagnostik and Therapieplanung." Dissertation, Technische Universität Berlin, 1988.

Appendix A 1

Viewing Station

Listing of jackets/folders
Single modality
Multimodality
Single image presentation   1024 x 1024 X ==> 12
Patient and image text
Control information acceptance and display   R
Contrast enhancement - windowing   R
4 - image presentation   512 x 512
Index presentation   64 x (64 x 64)
User ID, patient ID

Reporting Station

Listing and sorting of jackets
Multimodality
Imaging modality vs. organ based functions
Single image presentation   now 1024 x 1024 x 12
                                             1990's 2048 x 2048 x 12   R
Patient and image text   R
Conrol information acceptance and display   R
Indirect subimage contrast enhancement   (image buffer)
                                             (frame buffer)   R
window: CLAHE : unsharp mask   R
Index presentation simult w/   256 x (64 x 64)   R
   1 or 4/8 image presentation   4 x (1024 x1024)
                                             or 2048 x 2048   R

Zoom or Pan w/context overlay   (512 x512)   R
Listing and sorting of images in jackets   R
Annotation: test and overlay associated with image display
Static shaded - surface (colour)display   R
      w/superimposed (?) gray-slice (control of slice position)
2D vector graphic overlay colour, e.g. variable region of interest
(polygon)   R
Selection of image group via "alternator" or index   R
User ID, patient ID
Distance, angle and area measurements
Region of interest specification and measurements, average
      intensity   R
Memory requirements: 256 images à 12 bits;
                                             4 à 4096 x4096
                                             remainder à 512 x512

2 - image blinking

Cine
      2D
      2 1/2D
      3D
      Through rotation angles
      Through levels, e.g. iso-intensity levels
      Actual time sequences

High Capability Visualisation and Manipulation Station (HCVM)

2D Visualisation
All capabilities of reporting stations, except:
No fast alternator mode, no fast seledtion from index
Full parameter selection (CLAHE)   R
Object definition, as under 3D   R
Model-based computations, e.g. degree of deformation
Filtering -No?
3D Visualisation
Complex object display: rotation, scale   R
Multi object transparent display: transparency
    specularity and colour control, => 1 image source   R
    realistic display
Object definition - pointing: logical operations
    (union, difference, connected subregion)
Sculpting, image descriptor display ??   R
Object selection, removal   R
2D slice superimposition, dynamic selection   R
3D stereo and/or rocking. Parallaxis via head motion?   R
Landmark specification and deformation
Distance and volume measurement   seconds
Model - based computation (see 2D)
Image description and model preprocessing
Major computations done automatically
3D vector graphics -
    a) short term solution for surfaces
    b) for superimposition on shaded graphics

A comprehensive model for medical image data bases.

Y. Bizais, F. Aubry, B. Gibaud, J.M. Scarabin and R. Di Paola
Projet DIMI, University Hospital Nantes, France
Unité INSERM 66, IGR, Villejuif, France
Groupe SIM,University Hospital , Rennes, France
Groupe SIM, University Hospital ,Rennes, France
Unité INSERM 66, IGR, Villejuif, France

1 Introduction

Picture Archiving and Communication Systems (PACS) aim at providing an environment to store and retrieve medical images, and to distribute them. Several medical, technological and organizational problems must be solved before PACS can be introduced in clinical environments. In this paper, the specific features of (medical) images and their consequences on the development of Medical Image Data Bases (MIDB) are discussed. In particular we show that new conceptual solutions need to be found, if PACS are to provide more efficient ways of exploiting images.

In the first section, the need for highly structured MIDBs is shown, what cannot be achieved using classical data base management systems (DBMS). In the second section, basic approaches to develop MIDBs are discussed and our past experience in this field is outlined. Interestingly enough the three independent projects which are presented, conclude in the same way about the functional requirements and the possible solutions which can be used for developping efficient MIDBs. For these reasons a common project was defined and a working group (NRV-PACS) has been formed to realize it. This project is presented in the last section.

2 Do we really need MIDBs ?

This question can actually be broken into two parts :

1) Is it useful to store medical images digitally ?

2) If yes, do we need to develop special DBMSs for this purpose ?

It is considered that storing medical images in a digital way provides a *better and faster access* to them. However it is not clear that it is an efficient approach from an economical viewpoint, and some applications well-solved using films do not have a cost-efficient digital counterpart today (by instance, the distribution of images to clinics and wards). On the other hand *digital storing of medical images is a prerequisite to complex image processing* such as multimodality image processing or 3D image matching. Such techniques can be seen as better, more efficient ways of exploiting information present in medical images. We strongly believe that PACS can be accepted from medical and economical viewpoints, only if they provide some added value to medical imaging as we know it today. In other words PACS are viable only if they give easy access to sophisticated image processing techniques, which require the availability of MIDBs.

Consequently MIDBs able to handle generated data must be developed, as a key component of PACS. Can we develop such MIDBs using standard DBMSs ? The answer is no because, at each step of the management process, there are specific features of medical images which cannot be handled by such systems. Images are produced by acquiring and processing images: *the complex relationships existing between images*, image series and results *must be handled by the DBMS* as well as images themselves. Such relationships cannot be described using relational tools as we will show it later.

3 Some basic questions

To specify MIDBs it is necessary to answer basic questions about their potential use and architecture:

1) MIDBs can be made up of composite objects which can be retrieved but not updated. This is the standard viewpoint, for which PACS only provide digital means to archive and distribute medical images. in this case image retrieval and display is a digital analog of bringing a film onto a lightbox, and viewing it. On the other hand *MIDBs can be composed of updatable objects*, which are retrieved from the data base and from which new images are generated through image processing. The latter become new objects in the data base, and relationships to input images and image processing procedures must be kept as well.

2) MIDBs can be seen as a subsystem of acquisition devices, a key component of PACS (multimodality imaging) or a shared component of a HIS. It is our opinion that such *different MIDBs must have the same architecture to ensure compatibility and upgradability*. By instance an institution may start a PACS project by purchasing an image source equipped with a MIDB subsystem, and buy other sources and a communication system later. In fact this is the most probable approach to PACS and it requires the MIDB systems to be consistent. A common architecture is thus necessary.

3) MIDBs can be designed according to the ACR/NEMA standard or according to an *internal standard comprising the proper ACR/NEMA interfaces* for communication purposes. The last solution must be preferred because the ACR/NEMA standard is adequate to describe the transfer of images from a system to another one, but not to describe the internal organization of images.

In summary, our basic assumptions are:

1) MIDBs must be able to handle images and associated data produced by acquisition devices and image processing (updatable objects),

2) The various MIDBs (acquisition device subsystem, PACS component, HIS component) must share the same architecture,

3) MIDBs must strongly structure image information and provide ACR/NEMA interfaces for comunication purposes.

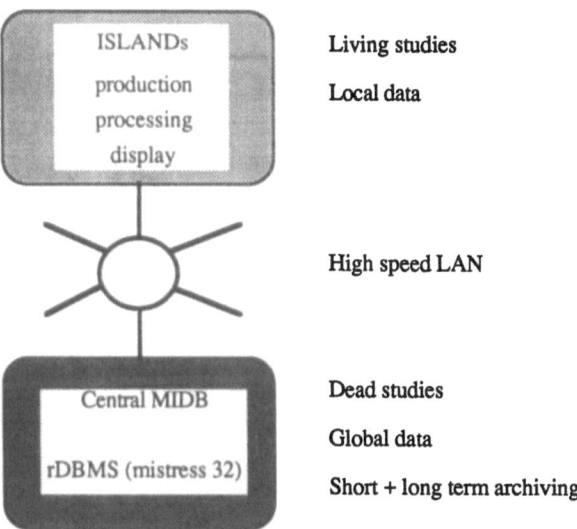

Living studies

Local data

High speed LAN

Dead studies

Global data

Short + long term archiving

Fig.1 : Architecture of the DIMI project system

4 Some tentative answers

4.1 The DIMI project (University Hospital of Nantes, France)

As shown in Fig.1 this prototype PACS system is made up of *several islands* (Unix running VICOMs) and a *central MIDB* (VAX 750), connected together through a high speed local area network.

In each island, images may be produced, processed and displayed. In most cases, images are produced and processed in the same island to minimize image transfer, but images can be imported from other islands for multimodality processing. Acquisition and processing procedures are predefined for each study. As long as all these procedures are not performed, the study is "living" and data are "local" (not accessible from outside). Then data are transferred to the central MIDB where they become "global".

Local and global MIDBs were designed using the same relational DBMS (Empress 32).

4.2 The SIRENE project (University Hospital of Rennes, France)

In this project *commercially available image sources* are connected to a *server* (Server 32, Copernique) and to a variety of *multimodality workstations* (RGN, faxicolor, telimage, sigma 200) through a local area network (matracom 6500), as shown in Fig.2. Image sources work independently and may send a selected subset of a study to the server in which they are reformatted. Afterwards archived images can be sent to the various workstations where they can be processed and displayed.

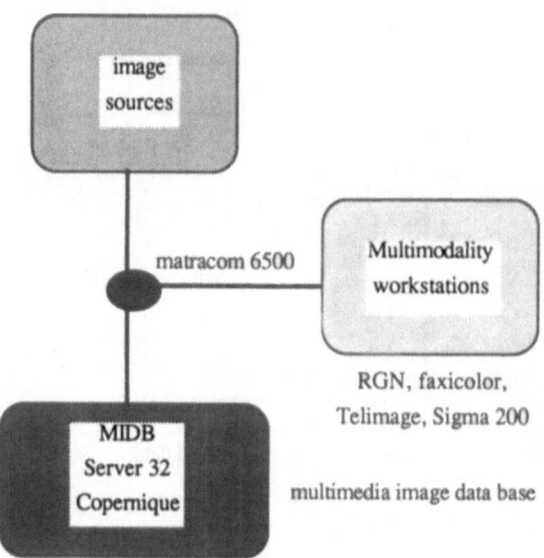

Fig.2 : Architecture of the Sirene project

The most interesting feature of this system is the MIDB system, which can handle multimedia data (text, image, voice) and communicate with other components through standard protocols.

4.3 The BDIM project (Inserm 66, Inst. G. Roussy, Villejuif)

It corresponds to the development of a MIDB subsystem for an MRI system, as shown in Fig.3. If this project is limited as far as the number of image sources is concerned, it is quite *ambitious in terms of MIDB functionalities*. It is based on Oracle (rDBMS), images and arrays are managed as generic items, an image query layer and an image processing interface were designed.

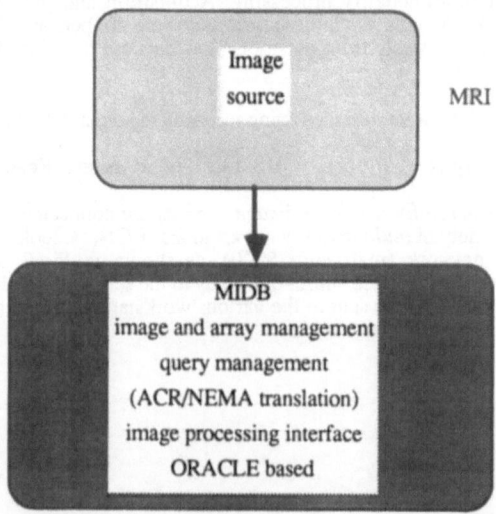

Fig.3 : Architecture of the BDIM project system
In fact this project can be seen as a first demonstrator of a true MIDB, as we defined it above.

4.4 What can be learned from these projects

1) each group started with quite a different view of what a PACS and a MIDB should be, and ends up with the same view (each system should include features of the two other systems to be satisfactory).

2) the three MIDBs are based on rDBMS which cannot describe image data and relationships properly.

3) the multimedia nature of medical image data, the complexicity of relationships between acquired and processed data require the development of new conceptual tools, before a usable solution can be derived. This is a far more difficult problem than that induced by the amount of data, for which a technological solution not specific to medical imaging must be found.

This is why we decided to join our efforts concerning MIDBs, a year ago, and formed the NRV PACS working group. In the following we define our main objectives and how we plan to achieve them.

5 The NRV-PACS MIDB project

5.1 Main objectives

We have four main objectives :

1) *to define the role of MIDBs within Health Information Systems*. Obviously medical images are one part of Medical Information and should be treated as such. Unfortunately, due to the specific nature of images, specific systems must be designed to handle such data. In a first step, it is thus necessary to define how images are produced and consumed to provide Health Information Systems with the proper links to such specific data management systems.

2) *to list objects to be managed by MIDBs*. Based on our previous experience we believe that the complex structure of image data must be understood clearly. For this purpose we plan to list image and associated data, allowed actions and authorized actors for as many studies as possible. This inventory will serve as a test data set for a global model.

3) *to model objects and to propose formal interfaces*. For all studies that we know the complex relationships between acquired and processed images cannot be described using relational tools. On the contrary, if it were possible to construct several levels of objects, then relationships would become clear, or at least their description would be simpler. Our preliminary work indicates that such an opportunity is offered by object-oriented tools. Such a model does not derive from the ACR/NEMA standard and consequently, interfaces must be designed to allow an object-oriented MIDB to communicate with other systems.

4) *to validate the model and to propose practical implementations*. It is clear that the object-oriented model is useful to describe image data, but that no object-oriented DBMS is available yet. It follows that practical and efficient solutions must be found to implement the proposed model.

5.2 Global structure of MIDBs

Due to the independent development of image sources, image workstations and medical data bases, the global information system cannot be based on a master/slave relationships, but rather on a distributed architecture.

Basically we think that MIDBs should provide the means *to store and access images and closely associated data*. Other data well-managed by standard DBMS and not required directly by image manipulation should be stored in connected systems such as RIS and HIS. It follows that MIDBs must include tools to describe images produced by image sources and image processing systems, as well as provide interfaces to such "data generating" systems and connected information systems. This global structure is shown in Fig.4.

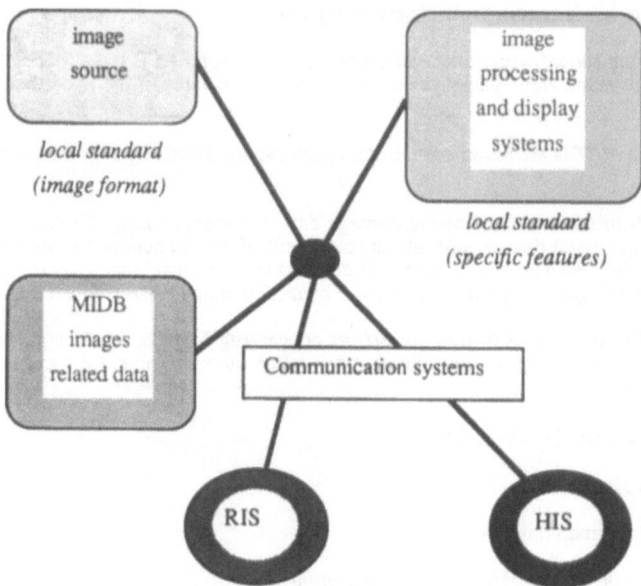

border-line items and connected systems

Fig.4 : Global structure of Medical Image Data Bases

Despite the apparent simplicity of this structure, it implies several fundamental consequences. Firstly the MIDB is seen as a *subsystem of the overall information system*, able to handle the specific nature of medical images. It means that we focus primarily on *image handling*, which has been neglected up to now. Secondly the MIDB does not belong to any specific component of the Health Information System, but have *privileged links with some components*. The reason for that is that some functionalities may involve only PACS components or even a single image source, while others make use of data stored in the MIDB and in other information systems. Such applications are beyond the scope of MIDBs and should be considered from a more general viewpoint.The development of MIDBs should be limited to providing tools to access image data because of its specificity.

5.3 Inventory of objects

As we said before a clear understanding of objects which are manipulated, and of relationships between objects is necessary. For this purpose, we propose to list objects and relationships for as many imaging procedures as possible. We do not expect to end up with a comprehensive inventory, but we hope to validate our model from it (see below).

For each *imaging modality*, there exists a limited number of *imaging procedures* (by instance brain scans and thoracic scans for X-CT). For each imaging procedure we plan to list :

1) *acquisition conditions* : how many images or image series are acquired, how images and image series are related, how images and series are characterized ...

2) *processing conditions* : how acquired images and image series are processed, in which ways acquired and processed images are related, how processed images and images series (eventually 3D data) are characterized ...

3) *display conditions* : how they can be characterized (specific features of workstations) ...

4) *miscellaneous* : which border-line objects (such as the report of a study) are generated and where they are kept, which connected systems (such as a RIS) are involved, which interfaces (to users, to networks, to image processing) are to be provided for such functions to be performed ...

We strongly believe that such an inventory will allow us to find numerous common *(invariant) features* among apparently different objects listed in the inventory. It will be then possible *to decribe objects in a unified fashion and to derive a compact model*.

5.4 Model design : interfaces

Two types of interfaces must be provided : user and system interfaces, and communication interfaces. When standard interfaces are available, they were analyzed and eventually selected to decrease development efforts and to provide the user with a standard environment.

For the *user level* we distinguish the following interfaces :

1) to workstations for which multi-windowing software such as X-window and further extensions are selected,
2) to image processing languages for which a specific development is required,
3) to query generation for which the query by example (QBE) and object-oriented (Hypertalk, Hypercard) approaches are evaluated,
4) for fuzzy and incomplete queries which are not considered in a first step.

The *system level* must take care of :

1) modifications of structure, to easily include new imaging procedures or new processing techniques,
2) data base consistency since object-oriented approaches do not have any mechanism to ensure it.

Finally *communication interfaces* must be included and the following solutions are considered :

1) standard interfaces such as OSI, TCP/IP and ACR/NEMA for common communication functionalities,
2) ODA for file transfer protocols,
3) an automatic translator is required to reformat image data coming from images sources and sent to workstations,
4) finally a specific image processing interface must be developped for the MIDB to communicate with image processing systems.

It can be seen that we put a *lot of emphasis on interfaces* for two main reasons :

1) the MIDB as we defined it above can only receive, store and send highly structured data.

Therefore comprehensive interfaces to systems producing images and to other information systems must be provided. Moreover the MIDB must take care of local formats used by image sources, image processing systems and workstations. Easy access to data from these systems is part of the data base design.

2) the complex structure of data and of their relationships makes it necessary to provide the user with proper interfaces to access data and to process them.

5.5 Model design : the object-oriented approach

Our previous experience shows that a true MIDB cannot be built on the basis of a relational DBMS. On the contrary *the object-oriented approach* exhibits several interesting features which makes it a good candidate to design a MIDB :

1) *Primitive types are flexible* such that images, arrays and ordered sets are easily represented.

2) *Such a model is "generative"* since object constructors (grammars) are available. It follows

that new object types can be defined easily, which is necessary since our inventory cannot be exhaustive, and since medical imaging is a rapidly expanding field. Moreover "actions on DB objects" can be described as "DB objects" themselves. Thus new actions can be defined as well. Finally evolution rules permit the upgrading of the data base while being consistent with data previously stored.

3) *Complex links between objects* are much better described than by using relational DBMS, through the concepts of aggregation, association, subclass and metaclass, and inheritence of properties. It is clear that such concepts find a direct use in the description of image series, or of the relationships between acquired and processed images.

However the object-oriented approach does not provide efficient tools to ensure DB integrity, consistency and security. Solutions to these drawbacks must be found since medical images are nothing else that medical information in this regard.

6 Model implementation and potential solutions

It is beyond the scope of this paper to describe how we plan to implement the above model. Nevertheless some indications must be given since no object-oriented data base management system is available yet.

If we go back to the classical vision of MIDBs, four layers can be distinguished :

1) the *patient layer* (type-1 items) which is fairly easy to model with rDBMS tools, and on which whole DB queries can be performed,

2) the *study layer* in which two types of items can be found : (type-2a) items well modelled by rDBMS tools and subject to whole DB queries (as patient items), and (type-2b) items describing the content of the study which are better described using object-oreinted tools, and are not subject to whole DB queries,

3) the *series layer* in which items (type-3 items) are similar to those of the second type in the study layer,

4) the *image layer* which is characterized by a large amount of data (type-4) to be managed by a filing system.

It follows that the object-oriented approach provides a neat way of describing the MIDB content (especially the complex relationships between images), but that a true object-oriented DBMS is not required to implement the model. More precisely a standard relational DBMS can be used to describe type-1 and type-2a items, while type-2b and type-3 items can be implemented as Lisp sentences stored as DB items and interpreted by ad hoc procedures. Other solutions such as SQL extensions and object-oriented systems are evaluated as well.

Therefore the complex model that we propose can be implemented and validated, even before a true object-oriented DBMS is available.

7 Conclusion

As a conclusion some provocative statements can be made concerning MIDBs to stimulate discussion on this wide-opened topic :

- the development of MIDBs is one of the most difficult task in building true and clinically efficient PACS.

- PACS will be successful only if MIDBs can manage images produced by image sources and image processing systems (added value to today medical imaging).

- MIDBs should not be seen as a PACS component only, but rather as a node able to store, receive and send data within a distributed system. More precisely it can be anything from a subsystem attached to an image source up to a system storing image in a Health Information System. In any case a common formal approach is necessary.

- MIDBs should only store images and data directly useful to image handling. Loosely associated data should be stored in other systems, with which MIDBs can communicate.

- Consequently MIDB developers should focus on image data modelling and (user and communication) interfaces.

- Relational DBMS do not constitute a good basis to develop MIDBs because their tools are too poor to describe the complex relationships between acquired and processed images. The object-oriented approach provides much more appropriate tools and should be considered as one of the solutions to develop MIDBs.

- Implementation of an object-oriented data model is difficult today, since object-oriented DBMS are not available. Nevertheless such a model can be validated by taking into account the specificity of the application.

References

De Valk J.P.J., Bakker A.R., Bijl K., Heijser W., Boekee D.E., Reijns G.L.: "PACS reviewed: possible and coming soon ?". *Journal of Medical Imaging*. 1987;1: pp 77-84

Assmann K., Venema R., Hoehne K.H.: "Software tools for the development of pictorial information systems in medicine : the ISQL experience". NATO ASI Series: *Pictorial Information Systems in Medicine*, HK Hoehne ed., Springer-Verlag, Berlin . 1986; pp 333-356

Zeleznik M.P., Maguire G.Q., Baxter B.: "PACS data base design". *SPIE* . 1983; 418 pp 287-295

Seshadri S.B., Khalsa S., Arenson R.L., Brikman I., Davey M.J. : "An image archive with the ACR-NEMA message formats". *SPIE* . 1988; Vol. 914;pp 1409-1415

Hachimura : "A prototype PACS with the capability of retrieval by image data", *CAR Proceedings*, Springer-Verlag, Berlin. 1987; pp 507-524

Renoulin R., Scarabin J.M. et al : "The Sirene project", *CAR Proceedings*, Springer-Verlag, Berlin . 1987; pp 525-531

Bizais Y., Baba-Ami M., Roy M., Martin E., Roy S. : "The DIMI project, an image processing and management computer facility for an imaging department". *SPIE* . 1986; 626:pp 656-663

Aubry F., Badaoui S., Kaplan H., Di Paola.R. : "A biomedical image data base : philosophy, design and implementation". 6th Europacs Conference, *Medical Informatics* 1988.

Medical Image Analysis, Storage, and Retrieval

Stelios C. Orphanoudakis
Institute of Computer Science. University of Heraklion PO Box 1385. GR-71110 Heraklion

In recent years, advances in computer science and engineering have resulted in significant developments in the field of medical imaging. New diagnostic imaging modalities produce digital images while conventional radiographic techniques are gradually being replaced by their digital counterparts. This has generated substantial interest in the development of integrated Hospital Information Systems which support the digital transmission, storage, retrieval, analysis, and computer assisted interpretation of distributed multimedia medical records consisting of textual, image, voice, and attribute data. The modeling and design of technically, conceptually, and functionally integrated Hospital Information Systems as well as the definition of requirements for the development of Picture Archiving and Communication Systems, which are properly integrated with other HIS components, are important technical challenges which must be met in the near future.

1 Introduction

The large number of medical images currently generated by different diagnostic modalities makes their routine handling and interpretation a very difficult task. The use of computer methods in the storage, retrieval, analysis, and interpretation of multimodality medical images is one of the major current trends in medical imaging [1]. This has been the result of an increased use of digital imaging techniques leading to a wide acceptance of computers and digital image processing techniques by the medical community.

Recent developments in x-ray computed tomography (CT), emission computed tomography (ECT), positron emission tomography (PET), digital radiography (DR), digital subtraction angiography (DSA), digital ultrasound, and magnetic resonance imaging (MRI) have paved the way for a filmless, digital Department of Diagnostic Imaging in the near future. The diagnostic imaging department of the future will make extensive use of computer networks, mass storage devices, and sophisticated workstations at which humans and machines will interact, assisted by techniques of computer vision and artificial intelligence, to achieve integration of multimodality imaging information and expert medical knowledge [2]. Computer networks will also provide physical links to other hospital departments and patient wards in order to improve inter-departmental communications and patient monitoring procedures. Picture Archiving and Communication Systems (PACS), supported by multimodality medical image databases, will also be integrated with all other components of a Hospital Information System (HIS). HIS integration must be achieved at a technical, conceptual, and functional level.

The purpose of creating an environment such as the one described above is to support medical decision making and integrated hospital care by improving communications and facilitating the acquisition, storage, retrieval, analysis, and interpretation of distributed multimedia documents (i.e. structured collections of attribute, text, image, and voice data [3,4]).

For the past two decades, the trend in medical imaging has been to probe the human anatomy and physiology using different types of energy and new methods of data acquisition and processing. The diagnostic imaging modalities which emerged as a result of related efforts have received a lot of publicity, but their true potential has not been fully realized. Specifically, the various medical imaging modalities collectively generate substantially more diagnostic information than that which is routinely extracted from visual displays and transcribed in medical reports. In order to improve the information transfer efficiency of medical imaging modalities or to minimize the loss of information between raw data acquisition and diagnostic interpretation, much work is needed in the area of computer-aided multimodality image analysis and interpretation. The integration of prior medical knowledge with information contained in multimodality image data and other components of a multimedia medical record is one of the major challenges facing humans and machines as they continue to become increasingly interdependent during the next decade.

Future efforts toward integrating computers into the diagnostic process should also address issues related to the design of intelligent medical imaging workstations. These workstations must allow the implementation and high-speed execution of image enhancement, restoration, analysis, and interpretation algorithms and must be capable of accomodating new advances in artificial intelligence and knowledge-based image analysis. Furthermore, they must support an intelligent man-machine interface which permits the retrieval of multimodality image data, the extraction of relevant diagnostic information from it, and its integration with prior medical knowledge, as this may be represented in human or machine memory.

The rate at which progress is made in providing computer-assisted integrated patient care will depend on further developments in the design and implementation of truly integrated HIS and PACS, which can handle distributed multimedia medical records efficiently, given the constraints of the real-time clinical environment. Rather than considering specific medical imaging and image analysis techniques, as they apply to medical imaging, in this short paper we consider the definition of requirements for the storage, retrieval, and general handling of distributed multimedia medical records in the environment of integrated distributed hospital information systems. Specifically, we consider issues related to the development and implementation of medical image databases as an important component of PACS, which is viewed in turn as an integral component of any HIS.

2 Integrated Hospital Information Systems

In this section, the key components of an integrated HIS are described and an architectural design which can be used to achieve system integration is proposed [5].

The main function of a hospital information system is to support the effective implementation of administrative and clinical activities. This is achieved by providing mechanisms for acquiring, storing, analyzing, and assisting with the interpretation of information which is considered important in clinical decision making. Such information and information management tools must be easily accessible by all authorized hospital personnel. Thus, a HIS provides channels of communication and workstations with built-in capabilities for information retrieval, analysis, and interpretation. The acceptability and acceptance of HIS by the medical community is highly contingent on user-friendliness and the degree to which data security can be guaranteed. [K

2.1 Components of a HIS

Based on the different clinical and administrative activities a HIS is required to support, it can be subdivided into the following [sub]systems:
1.   The Patient Information System (PIS). The PIS handles the entry, storage, and retrieval of all patient related data, provides access to a medical library, and facilitates the planning and control of patient flow through the hospital. Physically, it is a distributed data base system and its underlying conceptual organization is that of a hypertext [6]. The PIS should support the following tasks:
1)Creation and maintenance of complete patient records.
2)Picture archiving and communications (this is complementary to the previous task, but has unique technical requirements which must be taken into account in the design of the PIS).
3)Diagnostic reporting.
4)Planning and control of patient flow through the hospital.

2.   The Clinical Support System (CSS). The CSS consists of different [clinical] decision support [sub]systems whose function is to automate the well-structured, repetitive, often menial, and data intensive clinical tasks while enhancing physician skills in more challenging and creative tasks. The CSS can be implemented via a blackboard architecture [7,8], which consists of a blackboard, a language system, a knowledge base, a clinical problem processing system, and an explanation system.

3.   The Organizational Support System (OSS). The OSS supports administrative tasks such as billing, financial planning, planning and controlling of resources, etc. It must also provide the

required mechanisms to support adaptation to a changing health care environment (i.e. referal patterns, government imposed regulations, etc.).

4. The Communications System (CS). The CS provides real and elapsed time communication channels over which text, voice, and image data can be transmitted to support data and information exchange among the various departments of a hospital, between hospitals, or between a hospital and other health care providers.

Picture archiving and communication systems are embedded in and interact with all of the above components of a HIS and, therefore, are not listed as a separate component, although they have unique design and implementation requirements (see, for example, First International Conference on Picture Archiving and Communication Systems (PACS) for Medical Applications, SPIE, Newport Beach, CA, January 1982).

2.2 Architecture of an Integrated Hospital Information System

This section is concerned with the definition of an architecture for implementing the HIS components described previously. The proposed architecture is based on the assumption that the system must be decentralized, both in terms of where the data is stored and where the processing takes place. This is in agreement with current trends in HIS development and implementation [2]. A HIS implementation scheme which is based on a distributed architecture is not out of reach, considering recent advances in computer technology which have made a variety of powerful tools available at a rapidly decreasing cost (i.e. user-friendly workstations, domain specific software, distributed data base management tools, knowledge engineering tools, etc).

Coordinated decentralization is a prerequisite to achieving HIS integration. This in turn imposes certain requirements, which include:
1)A standardized operating system environment.
2)A standardized
classification of hospital divisions and their functions. It may also
be necessary to take into account established inter-departmental
information flow patterns.
3)A standardization of communication and networking protocols.
4)A consistent [and well defined] set of operational and procedural rules for governing hospital functions.

It is possible to achieve functional integration in a distributed HIS using a distributed blackboard architecture. Specifically, a HIS Administrator Blackboard can be implemented in the environment of the HIS data server to plan and control the functions of the HIS. To assist in this task, staff blackboards can be implemented, each of which specializes in the performance of certain functions such as scheduling of activities and resources, system planning, system monitoring, etc. The HIS Administrator delegates tasks to the PIS, CSS, OSS, or CS managing blackboards, receives status reports from them, and resolves conflicts which may arise in response to a certain inquiry.

The blackboard is a powerful metaphor, in which each of several HIS system components and subcomponents:
(1) take a turn considering the clinical support, or information processing, inquiry,
(2) consider how the inquiry may be satisfied, and
(3) return answers to the local blackboard, where they are examined and, if necessary, forwarded to the central blackboard. Depending on the nature of the inquiry, any blackboard can become central, i.e. plan and control activities posted on other (delegate) blackboards. Blackboards constitute expert system structures which provide intelligent support to HIS operations.

3 Medical Image Databases

An important problem in designing an integrated HIS is how to manage the large volume of image data. A variety of PACS configurations have been implemented and continue to be investigated in an attempt to find a good solution to this problem. However, one must also consider the design and implementation of properly indexed medical image databases or multimedia document bases, given that images are but one component of a multimedia medical record.

From the point of view of document retrieval, the various components of a multimedia document may be characterized as active or passive, depending on whether they can or cannot be used for accessing a document. To the best of our knowledge, only the attribute and text components are active in current multimedia document filing systems. In general, multimedia documents may be addressed by attributes or by content. The attribute (formatted) data are addressed using indexing techniques. The unformatted data consists of text, images (graphical and bitmap), and voice recordings. The textual content can be addressed using either indexing or other methods, such as signatures \cite{kn:Falo85}. The image and voice content is currently being addressed only indirectly, through associated text such as captions, or image/voice attributes (e.g. subject, speaker, etc.) [10,11].

The above situation appears to be the state of things in the area of office information systems, where the notion of a multimedia document as a basic entity has been developed. However, methods of image analysis have been used in different application domains to describe and model images and image classes, so that the content of particular images can be determined based on the correspondence between the derived description of a particular image and some appropriate model of an image class [12,13]. So far, most of the methods which have been developed are knowledge-based, making use of domain-specific knowledge, and are not particularly well suited for image retrieval by content and image data base work. This is primarily due to problems with computational efficiency, uncertainty, and general knowledge representation issues. Nevertheless, for certain medical applications, it should be possible to develop and implement techniques of image analysis, symbolic content representation, and modeling which can be used to store images efficiently and to retrieve multimedia documents by pictorial content.

Combining results from the areas of office information systems and image analysis is a natural next step and, indeed, efforts are already undertaken to integrate methods for addressing pictorial content into multimedia document filing systems. In the approach for addressing pictorial content discussed below, it is attempted to reduce the dependence on the application domain as much as possible; to provide a simple and fast indexing scheme; to ensure some tolerance to uncertainty with regard to image content; and to exploit all the associations of images with other document components.

In applying image analysis techniques to document retrieval by pictorial content, one must initially limit the search space, by considering well defined classes of pictures, and structure the corresponding model(s) in such a way that the matching process can proceed in stages. This is possible with hierarchical models or nested sets of models of increasing complexity and specificity. Matching with complex models is attempted only when matching with simpler models has has been achieved. Models of low complexity and specificity do exist, which are appropriate for a wide variety of picture description and retrieval by content tasks. Furthermore, in a top-down approach to model matching, the model may be used to guide the generation of appropriate picture descriptions. Another alternative is to combine top-down and bottom-up processes in order to avoid certain problems with uncertainty in hypothesizing the existence of a particular object in the picture on the basis of a model. Such problems are inherent in the top-down approach [14].

In multimedia document retrieval, even if a query is made by specifying pictorial content, it is the entire document which is accessed and not the contained image alone. This has important implications with respect to user-level operations and the design of a system to support them. In particular, there may be substantial uncertainty as to what the user is looking for and a query answer set may be enlarged due to inexact matching techniques. Consequently, query formulation ought to be iterative and flexible, enabling gradual resolution of user uncertainty, as well as associative, exploiting all possible associations between document components. Query formulation can be aided by imposing an organization on the available set of documents, using associations between document components, and browsing documents. Possible associations of images with other document components are: 1)Image to text, 2)Image to voice,and 3)Image to attribute: The images contained in a document belong to one or more image classes, characterized by image class attributes. Furthermore, attributes may be associated with single objects in an image.

A query on document pictorial content may specify:

a) The semantic content of an image. A range of options is available for specifying semantic content and accessing relevant images and the containing documents. Listed in order of increasing expected query processing time and expected number of false drops (i.e., documents included in the query answer set, which do not satisfy the query restrictions), these are:
1) Specify values of image semantic attributes. Access is made through indices stored in the image data base.
2) Specify associated text values, i.e. words or phrases contained in the image caption or in the main body of the text, where the image is referred to. Text access methods, such as signatures, are used here.
3) Specify the image or part of image sought by pictorial example. In this case, a sample image is furnished and the system has to analyze it, extract its semantic content, create an appropriate representation, and match this representation against the representations of images contained in the specified search space.
4) Finally, there is an option mentioned last not for its complexity but for being the least probable. This exploits a possible image to voice association, if a voice caption exists, by accessing the voice caption using text access methods.

b) The syntactic content of an image. Here, the positions of objects in an image are of interest. These are specified by pictorial example, as in (a3) above, and can be resolved using an indexing technique such as two-dimensional strings [15].

c) Various image features/primitives of image classes or particular objects contained in the image. These are specified as image attribute values and relevant images are accessed using indexing techniques.

d) Combinations of (a), (b) and (c).

When an image contains more than one objects, its structure is usually important in addition to the identity of the contained objects. This leads to queries on both semantic and syntactic content. At the query interface level, pictorial example is used combined with windows for specifying attributes and related text. Restrictions on image features, as in (c), are similarly accomodated.

A strategy was presented for addressing tne pictorial content of multimedia documents. In particular, semantic and syntactic content as well as other image features are addressed, associations of images with other document components are exploited, and user uncertainty is resolved by iterative and flexible query formulation. Methods developed on the basis of such a strategy will prove extremely important in the development and implementation of truly integrated HIS and PACS.

4 Conclusions

In this paper, we have simply outlined the requirements for the design and implementation of integrated distributed HIS and multimedia document bases, which can handle the analysis, storage, and retrieval of multimodality medical images as one of the components of a multimedia medical record. An architecture, based on distributed blackboards, has also been proposed for achieving technical, conceptual, and functional integration of HIS. PACS currently under development are viewed as an integral component of HIS, interacting with all other system components and supported by properly indexed multimodality medical image databases.

References

1) Orphanoudakis S.C..: "Supercomputing in Medical Imaging." IEEE *Engineering in Medicine and Biology*. December 1988;7 n°4, pp 16 -20.

2) Rennels G.D. and Shortliffe E.H..:" Advanced Computing for Medicine. Scientific American, 257(4): 154-161, October 1987.

3) Gibbs S., Tsichritzis D., Fitas A., Konstantas D., and Yeorgaroudakis Y.. *MUSE: A Multimedia Filing System*. IEEE Software. March 1987; 4, n°2, pp 4 -15,

4) Constantopoulos P., Orphanoudakis S.C., and E.Petrakis. "An Approach to Multimedia Document Retrieval on the Basis of Pictorial Content". Institute of Computer Science, Foundation of Research and Technology - Hellas, Technical Report RCC/CCI/TR/1988/011, March 1988.

5) Moustakis V.S., Orphanoudakis S.C.: "Requirements Definition for an Integrated Hospital Information System." Proceedings of the First European Conference on Information Technology for Organizational Systems (EURINFO '88), Athens, Greece, May 16-20, 1988. pp.852-858.

6) Conklin J.: " Hypertext: An Introduction and Survey." *IEEE Computer*, September 1987;.20 n°9, pp17-41.

7) Silverman B.G., Moustakis V.S..: "Expert System Issues in Innovator." In B.G. Silverman, editor, *Expert Systems for Business*, Addison-Wesley, Reading,Massachusetts, 1987.

8) Hayes-Roth F., Waterman D.A., Lenat D.B.: "An Overview of Expert Systems".In F. Hayes-Roth, D.A. Waterman, and D.B. Lenat, editors, *Building Expert Systems*, Addison-Wesley, Reading, Massachusetts, 1983.

9) Faloutsos C.: "Access Methods for Text." ACM Comp. Surveys. 1985; 17 n°1, pp 49 -74.

10) Christodoulakis S. et al.: "Multimedia Document Presentation, Information Extraction, and Document Formation in MINOS: a Model and a System." ACM Transactions on Office Information Systems. October 1986; 4 n°4.

11) Badal D.Z.: "MMFF: A Multimedia Forms Facility." IEEE Office Knowledge Eng.. 1987; 1, n°1 pp 3-17.

12) Rosenfeld A. and Kak A.C.: "Digital Picture Processing". Academic Press, New York 1982; 2.

13) Ballard D.H., Brown C.M.:. "Computer Vision". Prentice-Hall, Englewood Cliffs, N.J., 1982.

14) Nagao M. :"Control Strategies in Pattern Analysis". *Pattern Recognition*. 1984;17 n°1, pp 45-56.

15) Shi-Kuo Chang, Qing-Yun Shi, Cheng-Wen Yan: "Iconic indexing by 2-D strings." *IEEE Transactions on Pattern Analysis and Machine Intelligence*. PAMI-May 1987; 9 , n°3

PACS and HIS, a necessary and fruitful combination

A.R. Bakker

BAZIS, Central Development and Support Group Hospital Information System, Schipholweg 97, 2316 XA Leiden, The Netherlands.

1 Introduction

In this short paper first a global comparison is made of HIS and PACS. Next as the major reasons for coupling the systems are mentioned :
- the need for HIS data to be able to properly manage the image database
- the need to present images and alpha-numeric data together at the same   workstation.

Some information is given on the HIS / PACS coupling as realized within the Dutch PACS project.

2 Comparison of HIS and PACS

The concept PACS and HIS are almost identical. Both systems are aiming at :
- coherent storage of data from different sources in a "central" database
- make data available to **authorized** users at the moment they are needed, at the location where needed and in a presentation adapted to the needs of the users.

  Despite this similarity in concept the practical realizations are quite different. To understand this it is worthwhile to notice that there are significant differences in relevant system parameters.

	HIS	PACS
Types of data	Alpha -numeric	Pictures
Size of records	100 - 200 Bytes	1-6 MBYTES
Number of records types	Hundreds	Dozens
Range of applications	Wide	Limited
Data acquisition	Manuel	Automatic (scanning,direct connection of modalities)

The recent IMIA working conference "Towards New Hospital Informatique Systems" stated : "PACS is logically to be considered as a subsystem of HIS

3   HIS and PACS different markets

HIS and PACS are presently dealing with quite different types of application and different classes of users within the hospitals. If we look at the market we can observe that HIS development is mainly carried out by :
- dedicated system houses
- cooperating groups of hospitals
- main computer manufacturers.

The development of PACS on the other hand is mainly carried out by suppliers of imaging modalities and by large research institutions.

We can observe that till now too little atttention has been paid to the relation between PACS and HIS. The synergetic effects that might be archieved have not been realized yet. This is probably caused by the different orientation of the suppliers of the systems.

4   Image storage in PACS

For the realization of a storage structure with sufficient capacity on one hand and acceptable performance on the other hand a multi layered structure is proposed.
-       The lowest layer is the archive containing all images. Such an archive should have a huge capacity (at least several Tera bytes). As technology we can think of   juke boxes of optical discs. At this moment the access time is rather long,   especially when a disc has to be loaded.
-       At the next level we find the central buffer holding images with an increased   probability to be needed. The typical capacity of the central buffer will be 10 to 100 gigabytes. At this moment Winchester technology seems most appropriate.
-       The top level is a localbuffer within the workstation holding the image under s t u d y .   T h e capacity will be approximately 100 megabytes directly addressable.

To be able to realizee acceptable response times even in this architecture an algorithm for prefetching of the images is needed.

5   Prefetching algorithm

The buffer works more or less as a cache for the archive. Apart from the similarity with cache memories for main computer memories the following differences should be mentioned :
-       Because of the "locality" of memory references in main computer memory, the   cache is in general loaded passive. In our PACS we can not expect such a "locality"   so an active algorithm is necessary to perfetch images.
-       Because of the large number of memory references to the cache of main memory in computers a miss in general is not a problem, since by averaging in performance improvement is significant. In a PACS the number of references to images is   limited, so a small nuber of misses can already lead to unacceptable response time.
-       The ratio between access time are different for the main memeory cache and the   buffer   / archive combination.

In a prefetching algorithm the following parameters can be expected to play a role :

- **Image related parameters :**
. type of examination (RIS)
. requesting specialism (RIS)
. date of examination (RIS)
. report of examination (RIS)
. status of examination (RIS)
. previous use of image (?)

- **Patient related :**
. admitted (HIS)
. on waiting list and planned data of admission (HIS)
. current appointment for outpatient wards (HIS)
. current appointment for radiology department (HIS)
. diagnosis (HIS)
. treating specialisme (HIS)

From this list of relevant parameters it is obvious that a coupling of HIS / RIS and PACS is essential for feeding a prefetching algorithm.

6   A possible prefetching algorithm

The following simple algorithm migth lead already to significant improvements of performance. The algorithm is different for inpatients and outpatients.
For inpatients activate the following images :

- most recent version of an examination plus one older version if the result is abnormal
- load examinations ordered by other specialisms only if these are not older than N1 month
- don't activate images automatically that are older than N2 months.

For outpatients :
- activate only images of the treating specialism
- activate only the most recent version plus one older if the result is abnormal
- don't activate images older than N3 months.

7 PACS / HIS coupling in the Dutch PACS project

Within the Dutch PACS project three phases of HIS / PACS coupling are foreseen:
- Phase 1: Coupling of the BAZIS HIS with the Philips Marcom prototyper at the   Utrecht University Hospital. Only data flow from HIS towards PACS.
- Phase 2 : Bidirectional coupling of BAZIS HIS and Philips Marcom prototype.
- Phase 3 : General HIS / PACS coupling.

At the moment phase 1 is operational in the Utrecht University Hospital. Within this phase by means of o PC based protocol converter the following events are signalled from HIS to PACS :
- admission of a patient to the ward where the clinical evaluation of PACS in being carried out
- discharge fromp ward
- appointement made for the radiology department
- appointement for the radiology department changed
- appointement at the radiology department cancelled
- radiology report authorized.

All messages from HIS to PACS are in ACR / NEMA format.

The data transmitted are used for patient identification and for display of reports. At present the data are not being used yet for improvement of the image management software.

Computer-Assisted Radiology: RIS / PACS
Attemps at Definition and Questions of Interfacing

K. Retter, A.J. Herbst, O. Rienhoff
Medizinische Informatik, Philipps Universität. D-3550 Marburg

Die Schwierigkeiten der Abgrenzung von Systemen wie RIS und PACS stehen in Kontrast zu den vermeintlichen Komplettlösungen in den Broschüren manncher Hersteller. In der vorliegenden Arbeit werden diese Diskrepanzen beleuchtet und die Notwendigkeit zur Aufarbeitung des Themas begründet. Das in Marburg entwickelte Drei-Sichten-Model könnte zu einer Strukturierung des Problems beitragen.

The difficulty to differentiate between RIS and PACS is in contrast to apparently comprehensive solutions painted by some manufacturers in their brochures. In the following presentatin these discrepancies are brought to light and the necessity to analyse this situation is justified. A methodology developed in Marburg may provide the basis for a useful solution.

1. Attempts at definition and problems of scope

Definitions of Radiological Information Systems (RIS) and Picture Archiving and Communication Systems (PACS) are needed in order to discuss the question of interfacing them sensibly. A likely approach may be based on the usage of the acronyms RIS and PACS and the historical development of these concepts.

A RIS is an information system for a radiological department. As is the case with any other information system (xIS) the purpose of a RIS is to comprehensively support information use in the department. Because this information is used for the organization or management of the department the terms radiological operations system (ROS) (1) or information management system (RIM) (2) are also used. The functional spectrum supported includes :

. Patient identification   . Billing support
. Request registration   . Film tracking and archiving
. Scheduling   . Enquiry functions
. Examination documentation   . Management information
. Report writing   . Research support

Additional system functions include the ability for customization and the normal system maintenance functions. Historically these systems are based on the one hand on the recording of service units (examinations) for billing purposes or report generation and, on the other, on text processing systems for reporting. In general RIS systems do not process radiological images, but provide film tracking and archiving functions and in cases include references to digital image stores (3) or digitally controlled film roll archives (4).

One of the first ideas to communicate and archive radiological digital images originated approximately six years ago (5). The "First International Conference and Workshop on Picture Archiving and Communications Systems (PACS) for Medical Applications" in 1982 created a forum for the discussion of this theme and at the same time coined the acronym PACS (6,7). In the mean time expectations have grown, and the ideal PACS is commonly understood to be a system with a fast LAN across which various image generating equipment can interactively send image data which is then stored in a central archive from which the images may be retrieved for viewing and manipulation on distributed workstations. In addition both hard copy and film digitizers are part of an ideal PACS (8,9,10,11,12,13, 14,15,16). In fact this system has so far only been realized in the glossy broschures of the manufacturers.

In contrast to the above mentioned acronym RIS, the acronym PACS is used for a variety of systems handling radiological images. In subsequent developements the comprehensive PACS has to a large extend made way for so- called "bottom- up" approaches (17). :

a. Teleradiography, or the communication of images over long distances to share interpretation facilities.

b. Linking image generating equipment, for example linking CT equipment of two sections to create the opportunity for cooperation interpretation.

c. Image presentation, in order to view and compare from two or more modalities, for example CT and DSA;

d. Quantitative image evaluation, especially in the case of digital radiography, presents an interesting possibility. In this case the acronym PACS may also stand for "Picture Analysis and Communication Systems" (18).

e. Image post-processing, where the emphasis is on image processing, for example 3-D reconstruction or animation studies.

f. Digital Archive. In view of the legal requirements for the long term storage of X-ray images and the subsequent storage, staff and film costs hopes of a solution in the from of digital archives have been raised. This solution, however, lead to a number of further requirements which bring it close to the ideal PACS sketched earlier.

On conferences like CAR (Computer-assisted Radiology) (11,12) this multiplicity of approaches are amply illustrated, little is said about RIS, even though these systems supposedly assist radiology. For approaches such as the latter the question of interfacing at the functional and data level of RIS and PACS systems cannot be ignored. In this case a knowledge of the boundaries of these systems is essential. But even this is problematical, even if only one of the above approaches is chosen.

2. The need for a solution

The differentiation between RIS and PACS may be due to functional differences, but could simply be the result of the different state of development between the two kinds of systems. For the remainder of the discussion it doesn't matter whether one sees it as two aspects of the same system, or as two separate systems. In other words, whether we are talking about *integration* or *interfacing*.

Independent of the chosen PACS-variant, at least as far as patient identification is concerned, common or redundant use of information with a RIS will result. The archive administration will require a functional differentiation between PACS and RIS. Additionally it will cause problems to assign the information created and used during the process of image generation up to image interpretation unambiguously to RIS or PACS. To complicate the matter further the problem of PACS-RIS cooperation is not totally divorced from the question of RIS-HIS coupling (19).

In view of the heterogeneous PACS solutions and the different stages of development in the market, the problem of differentiation should be solved by analysis of the application domain. Otherwise one runs the danger of fitting the problem to the tool, instead of the tool to the problem. The current PACS development is at a stage where such consideration may still be included in the development process.

3. The Marburg Methodology

The Marburg model was developed to statisfy the need for a powerful description of the radiological environment to act as a basis for the specification of an interface between RIS and PACS systems from different vendors. During the derivation of the model it became clear that various representations or "views" of the radiological environment would be needed. Three views were chosen, namely functional, control and data views. The views are depicted graphically to enhance communication between the model developers themselves and radiological personnel.

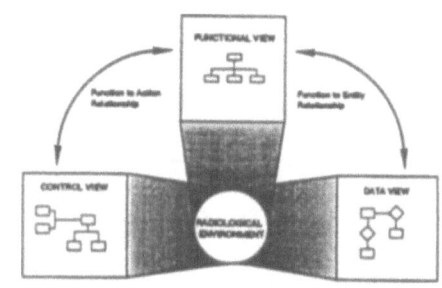

Figure 1. The three views of the Marburg Methodology.

The starting point of the model is a hierarchical breakdown of the functions in the radiological environment. The radiological environment includes the function of requesting the service (including the final report to the requestor). The hierarchical nature of this functional view allow us to develop the model for a specific case.

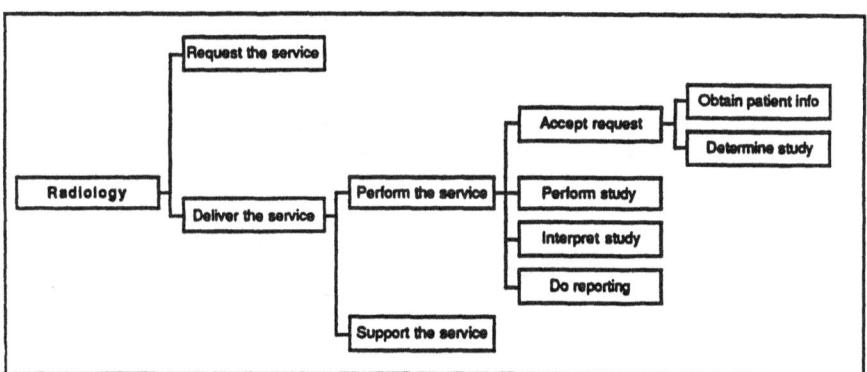

Figure 2. An extraction from the hierarchy of functions in a radiological environment as described in [21].

It has become clear through the use of various other system analysis methodologies that the inclusion of temporal aspects in the analysis of medical processes is crucial (20). The temporal aspect of the model is provided by the second or flow of control view. This view is represented by a state transition network, showing how the execution of actions cause the transition from one state to another. We have extended the state transition paradigm to include the ability to show decision points as well as the requirement that various states should be reached before a subsequent action may take place.

RIS and PACS systems are information systems, with the storage and communication of information central to their function. The structure of this information is described in the third view by an entity-relationship model.

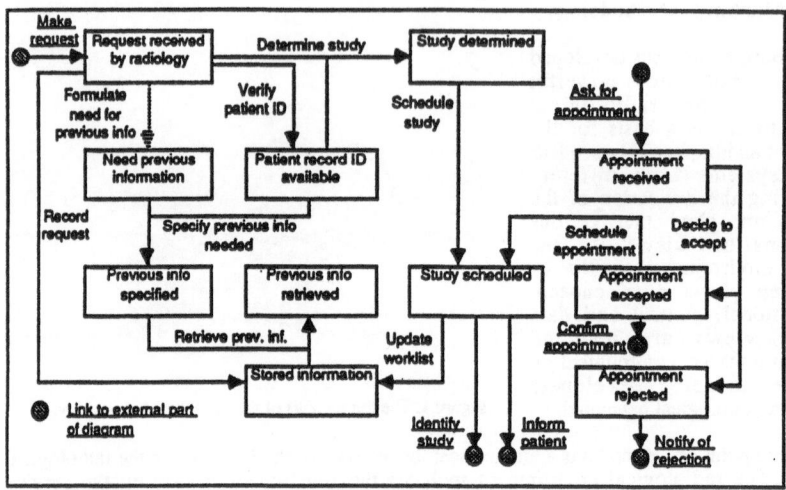

Figure 3. Flow of control at radiological reception as described in [21].

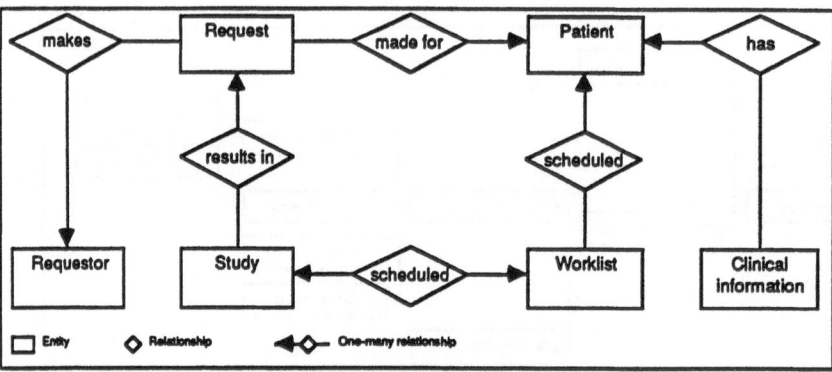

Figure 4. Part of the entity-relationship diagram as described in [21].

The most important characteristic of the model however is the way in which the views are related to one another . This enable the views to function as a coherent whole, as well as providing the opportunity to check that the views are consistent with one another . A table shows the relationship between the views. A function on the lowest level of the functional hierarchy is related to one or more actions which make up the function in the control view. A function is also related to the data view by specifying the entities used as input and output by the particular function.

A description of the methodology used to derive the model is beyond the scope of this presentation and will be described in a later publication (21). When interpreting the examples it should be noted that due to limited space the windows on the different views of the model do not coincide completely.

After the model is completed a specification of the interface between specific RIS and PACS systems may be derived in the following fashion. In view one each function is allocated to RIS, PACS, both, or neither of the two systems. Using the table relating a function to actions, each action is further classified as belonging to PACS or RIS. In view two the states which are preceeded and succeeded by actions belonging to different systems are marked. The marked states represent control points in the communication between the RIS and PACS systems. The entities or data structures involved in this communication may be derived by relating the action to the function it belongs to, and back via the table to the entities used as input and output by this particular function.

Once the interface points have been derived the actual interface protocol may be defined on the application level of the ISO layered model.

4. Discussion

The Marburg methodology is related to the SADT methodology used by Peccoud (22,23), but incorporates an entity-relationship model as an integral part of it, as opposed to using the IDA methodology to provide this capability . Petri nets are not used in the second view because of the difficulty to represent decisions in this formalism (24). The functional view provides it with a level of generality which is difficult to achieve in the data flow approach such as used by Simen (1). Our approach has many aspects in common with the information flow analysis used at the University of North Carolina (25,26), but distinguish it from their approach by the incorporation of an explicit data model, a generalized functional model, and a specific methodology to derive a PAC-RIS interface specification. During the initial phases of developing the model we tried to incorporate functional temporal aspects in one diagram, in a similar way to the SADT methodology, but found that we often emphasized the one to the detriment of the other.

In the use of this methodology during the past year it has greatly facilitated the communication between RIS and PACS developers as well as radiologists. It provided a common conceptual framework which the various developing teams have used as a basis in their design discussions. It resulted in specific changes in system design due to the fact that previously implicit assumptions have made way for more explicit understanding due to constructing the model. Beside these "side-effects" the interface specifications derived from the model at this point are comprehensive and directly usable in the system engineering effort.

It is hoped that this model may contribute to the ACR:NEMA (27) efforts in standardizing the RIS/PACS interface, or for an integrated approach to radiological information management.

Bibliography

1) Simen D.C., Sherman A.B., Edelstein S.A.. "Radiology: A communications view.". In (15) pp 686-687.

2) Retter K.: "Aspekte der Bildbeschreibung." In (13) pp 129-139.

3) Tiemann J.: "Grundlagen der digitalen Radiographie - Probleme der speziellen Datentechnik." in (12) pp 26-35.

4) Rienhoff O.: "Originalbild-, Microfilm- und digitale Archivierung - Übersicht und aktueller Stand". in (13) pp98-104.

5) Maguire G.O.: "Looking back at PACS attempts - What has happened since PACS I, in (9) pp 319- 400.

6).Schneider R.H., Dwyer S.J. (eds): 1st International Conference and Workshop on Picture Archiving and Communication Systems (PACS) for Medical Applications. *Proc. SPIE* 318. The International Society for Optical Engineering, Bellingham 1982.

7) Greinacher C.F.C., Fuchs D., Müller K.. "PACS: ein Zukunftsthema wird Gegenwart." *Electromedica* 1985; 53 (3) pp 96-103.

8) Greinacher C.F.C, Müller K., Fuchs D.: "Digitale Bildinformationssysteme in der Radiologie - Stand und Entwickelungstendenzen"

9) Höhne K.H.: "Digital Image Processing in Medicine" Proceedings, Hamburg October 1981, in: *Lecture Notes in Medical Informatics* . Springer Verlag, Berlin Heidelberg New York, 1981; 15.

10) Höhne K.H.: "Pictorial Information Systems in Medicine." NATO Advanced Science Institutes Series, Series F: *Computer and Systems Science* Springer Verlag, Berlin Heidelberg New York Tokyo,1984; 19.

11) Lemke H.U., Rhodes M.L., Jaffee C.C., Felix R. (Eds) "Computer Assisted Radiology". Proceedings of the International Symposium CAR 85 in Berlin, Spring Verlag, Berlin Heidelberg New York Tokyo, 1985.

12) Lemke H.U., Rhodes M.L., Jaffee C.C., Felix R. (Eds) "Computer Assisted Radiology." Proceedings of the International Symposium CAR 87 in Berlin, Springer Verlag, Berlin Heidelberg New York, 1987.

13) Riemenn H.E., Kollath J.: "Digitale Radiographie- Referate und Vorträge 1." Frankfurter Gespräche über Digitale Radiographie 1984 in Bad Nauheim. Schnetztor-Verlag, 1985.

14) Riemann H.E., Kollath J., Rienhoff O.: "Digitale Radiographie - Referate und Vorträge, 2." Frankfurter Gespräche über Digitale Radiographie 1986 in Bad Nauheim. Schnetztor- Verlag, 1987

15) Schneider R.H., Dwyer S.J. (eds): "Picture Archiving and Communication Systems (PACS III) for Medical Application." *Proc of SPIE.* . The International Society for Optical Engineering, Bellingham 1985; 536.

16) Schneider R.H., Dwyer S.J. (eds): "Picture Archiving and communication Systems (PACS IV) for Medical Applications." *Proc of SPIE.* The International Society for Optical Engineering, Bellingham 1986; 626..

17) Van Erning L.J.Th.O., Bongers P.A.G., Rothuizen P.: "PACS in practice: Software linking as a first step." In (11) pp 496-506.

18) Picture *Analysis* and Communication Systems

19) Rienhoff O., Retter K., List E.: "PACS and HIS -A difficult marriage." In (12) pp 493- 495.

20) Rolland C., Bodart F., Leonard M.: "Temporal Aspects in Information Systems", *IFIP*. North Holland, Amsterdam. 1988.

21) Greinacher C.F.C, Herbst A.J., Ihringer M., Prior F., Retter K., Rienhoff O.: "A General PACS-RIS Interface- An Analytical Approach to Information Use in Radiology". To be published as part of " Lecture Notes in Medical Informatics" Springer Verlag Berlin Heidelberg New York 1988.

22) Cinquin P., Demongeot J., Chbre-Peccoud M., Giraudin J.P.: "Specification of an integrated hospital information system with computer- assisted information system design methods." MIE 87. EFMI Rome 1987, pp31-35.

23) Chabre-Peccoud M., Cinquin P., Demongeot J.: "Modelling and Simulation of HIS." *Proceedings of "Towards New Hospital Information Systems"* IMIA Nijmegen 1988.

24) Peimann C.J.: "Modeling Hospital Information systems with Petri Nets." *Methods of Information in Medicine* . 1988; 27 pp17-22.

25) Rogers D.C., Wallace R., Thomson B.G., Parrish D.M.: "Information flow analysis as a tool for PACS development." In (15) pp 690-697.

26) Parrish D.M., et al: "Functional requirements for interfacing PACS to RIS." In (15) pp 597-601.

27) Digital Imaging and Communications. ACR-NEMA Standards Publication No 300-1985. NEMA 1985.

Some experience from a PACS-prototype in the Karolinska Hospital Stockholm, based on the "open system " principle.

Roger R. Gullquist
Stockholm County Council, Medical Informatics P.O. Box 9099, S-10272 Stockholm Sweden

Background

Digital principles in medical imaging has been used for almost twenty years in clinical practice and an increasing number of imaging modalities takes the advantage of digital signal processing.

This development is going on continuously with better diagnostical and treatment opportunities as a consequence.

The amount of information created for helping medical professionals to make adequate decision has rised enormously during the last decades and has come to a point where it is almost impossible to manage all information procuded. We are living in an era where we must find new technologies for managment of all information we have struggled for the created and medical images does stress this statement much do to the huge amount of data connected with digital images. PACS has become a very central tropic the recent years because it deals with the problem how to manage large data volumes.

Many vendors have been talking about PACS for some years but very few pratical implementations have been done in our hospitals.

At the Karolinska hospital there was a early interest of PACS but it was also obvious that many problems were to be solved before one could take advantage of the technology. Beside pure technical problems like storage capacity, image transfer velocity, image workstations and so on there are many other problems related to organizational aspects, educational aspects and not least financial aspects.

The Stockholm County Councils and the Karolinska hospital decided to build a PACS prototype at the Karolinska hospital with financial support from the Swedish federation for county councils, not because it should solve the actual problems with the managment of images, but to learn what king of problems arise when PACS technology is introduced in a hospital.

In Sweden there is a great interest to develop "open systems" which means that a PACS structure must be able to handle equipment from different vendors and a common image archive should be based as far as possible on industrial standards .

The PACS prototype

A Swedish company in the field of medical imaging, Imtec Inc. in Uppsula, was engaged to install a fibreoptic network call "Imnet" and appropriate interfaces to four digital image-sources, Siemens MR, Toshiba CT and Acuson ultrasonic scanner was constructed. An image workstation called "Epsilon" with a limited magnetical disk archive was connected to the network in order to evaluate the clinical images from different images sources. The hospital local area network "KS-net" which is ethernet-based, was also connected with the image workstation and the Siemens CT and MR in order to study a parallel network solution.

Conclusion

The overall most cumbersome work was to establish appropriate interfaces to the different image-sources due to lack of standards in many levels.

The Siemens CT and MR was quite easy to interface because they use common used computer architecture with well known interfaces.

The Toshiba CT was very difficult to interface according to the more "closed" computer architecture and it ended with central negotiations with Toshiba in order to get information on how to interface it to the network.

A general problem was also the different formats of image and administrative data in the digital image sources, it was necessary to reformat the data before storing them in the archive.

The performance in image transfer in the "Imnet" network was better for high volumes if images tranferred at a limited time periode (at the most 5-10 times) in comparison with ethernet. On the other hand was the ethernet performance better at single image transfers due to the "overhead" in the Imnet-protocol.

When loading a network with much traffic the Imnet performance is expected to be better than the ethernet because of the exponentially rising (collisions) time in ethernet protocol.

The great advantage of ethernet is doubtless the standardization (ISO8802.3) which means widely spread products and easyness to connect new devices. The draw-back of the Imnet is the lack of standard and the request for special interfaces.

The Epsilon workstation was excellent with respect of userinterface and monitor quality and was quick accepted by the medical professionals.

The draw-back was again the lack of standard with respect to the operating system, and the possibility of using standard video output for hardcopy.

A common problem is also the lack of standard in the area of PACS-RIS interface, a problem outside this prototype project but the effect of the absence of PACS-RIS integration was obvious in the use of the PACS prototype.

Multidimensional Image Modelling

F. Beltrame, P. Morasso, C. Ruggiero, G. Sandini, V. Tagliasco
DIST - University of Genoa, ITALY

The recent developments of medical technology have made it possible to investigate physiological system and organs to a much greater extent in the last few years. Specifically, a much better knowledge of the shape of human organs in normal and pathological conditions has been achieved, but often the rendering modality of anatomical structures is quite different from the one deriving from "normal" anatomy. An example is given by computer tomography, representing sections of human body, that is making available most valuable clinical information with presentation modalities different from the ones familiar to clinicians. Other cases in which a reexamination of the modalities of presenting anatomical structures may be required are: MRI, US, nuclear medicine. Linking the new technologies with pre-existing medical knowledge is becoming increasingly important, as long as new investigation techniques give access to valuable information. Medical imaging is perhaps the most striking example of this, but similar problems also arise - as a consequence of technology advances -.in other cases of medical data measurement, such as biomedical signal analysis, a field in which the possibility of routine ambulatory recording and multichannel recording has reduced in some cases the importance of longitudinal, time limited signal recording for medical diagnosis.

The proposed project aims to achieve a reformulation of medical knowledge in which human body segments are characterized by their 3-D shape as obtained from imaging methods.

As refers to 3-D representation and modelling of body segments, it is intended to use techniques to create solids starting from tomograms, for 3-D regionalization and contour following, and techniques for deformation of solids, such as tensorial calculus and spline based surface modelling.

1 Multidimensional Model Guided Image Interpretation

The field of matching iconic image information with labeled models in databases is one of the fastest growing fields in image processing and pattern recognition. Methods to be applied for the solution are developed not only in application to medical problems, but also in remote sensing, robot-vision, automated vehicle guidance, cognition, etc..

The automatic tracking and delineation of complex structures is a very important task in medical images, but to date techniques have relied on simple methods to segment the image data. For example, thresholding to determine bone structures in X-ray CT or the use of implicit models and special rendering techniques to display the surface of some soft tissue structures (Hohne et al. 1988).
There also has been considerable work on the display of 3D structures and surfaces, usually after substantial effort by an operator to hand-segment the image or with the use of local segmentation rules (Herman et al. 1988).
Finally, there is a number of published papers considering the problem of fitting arbitrarily complex biological shapes and providing algorithms to fit to any given outline or surface (Terzopoulus et al. 1988, Sequira 1987). In all these cases, the underlying model of the biological structure and the imaging system is implicit in the segmentation and tracking process. The model-guided matching techniques proposed here should build on these methods but with the requirement that the structure and imaging models are made explicit, and the matching techniques should be general purpose, with tuning for a specific image and modality. Important components of such a system are:

1) generation of special matched filters from stored models
2) optimization techniques for matching structures in images (e.g.

linear/ dynamic programming, relaxation)
3) confidence and goodness-of-fit measures
4) geometric constraint management
5) complex shape descriptors
6) feedback.

2 Multidimensional Modelling

Although the data acquired by CT, NMR or PET are inherently three dimensional, they have traditionally been visualized as a series of two-dimensional slices. Methods are now evolving that permit the entire 3D data set to be presented for display or interaction, through reprojection (Harris et. al. 1979), multi-planar reconstruction (Glenn et. al. 1975), or shaded surface display. Furthermore the clinical validity of of these 3D displays is beginning to be established (Burk et. al.). Preparing shaded surface display of from full-resolution medical data sets require massive computations.

Software system for this purpose are, thus, very slow typically taking several minutes to generate an image on the kind of machines used to acquired the raw data. This precludes any possibility for interactive operation. While programmable graphic processors (Fuchs et. al.) and special purpose hardware have been used to generate such images, non of the systems have the computational power to produce real-time real-time update to operator requests. Real-time update is particularly critical for those functions which are naturally controlled by graphics input devices. The need for special purpose hardware capable to achieve these performance is now clear. It is worth noting that the kind of special purpose hardware which is commercially available now (like for example the Silicon Graphics 4D/60, or the HP 350Srx Workstations) are all "rendering oriented" and for these reason they base the real-time performance on surface models of the object. The time necessary to produce such models from series of slices is still the significant part. It is obvious then, that, if the interactive operation involves the modification of the solid model, not only the rendering time must be considered but also the time necessary to modify the model. It is now clear that in order to provide a wide variety of 3D display alternatives including shaded surfaces, arbitrary reslicing, and (ultimately) the display of 4D databases a different approach must be followed.

Among the few architectures proposed, the one which has been developed more is that developed at the University of Pennsylvania by the group of Samuel Goldwasser (1984, 1986). The architecture provides the real-time display and manipulation of a 64x64x64 sub-volume of a 3D medical data set, with 4 bit-planes allowing 16 density levels. Future (and may be realized now) prototypes will be 256x256x256x16. Interactive features include: windowing, rotation, scaling, and slice planes. The 3D real-time Physician's workstation build around this voxel processor is composed of four hardware components (a host computer (VAX), a 3D Voxel Processor Prototype, a 2D frame buffer and an interactive control panel) and four software components (preprocessing utilities, volume of interest extraction, voxel processor control and off-line image generation).

3 Project Workplan

3.1 Multidimensional Model Guided Image Interpretation

The study will be organized in three sections:

- collection and discussion of existing methods
- definition of tasks to be solved for a successful combination process
- evaluation and tests of new developed methods.

Types of image material intended to start with will be:
- X-ray images
- CT-scan
- MR-scan.

The development in the area of model-guided image interpretation will be primarily software methods and techniques. The results or deliverables will be technical reports, computer code and demonstrator systems. The evaluation of the results will take a number of forms:

1) phantom-image trials - testing the techniques on "phantom" images designed to test specific aspects, e.g. resolution and noise response,
2) real-image trials - testing the methods against a database of correctly segmented images and measured parameters,
3) expert assessment - advice from clinicians etc.,
4) Monte Carlo simulation - test the robustness of the system within the assumed imaging models.

3.2 Multidimensional Modelling

Multidimensional Modelling is the driving aspect of the project: being able to model, represent and display objects in 4D (i.e. solid objects whose shape changes dynamically). As it was outlined in the status of the art part of the proposal, this topic has not received, up to now, the adequate attention probably because of the hardware limitations inherent in the class of machines used to acquire and process biomedical data.

Among the characteristics that will be taken into account regarding the modelling techniques, the most important are:

- Accessibility. The representation used by the modelling part should be based on features that are reasonably achievable from real data.

- Congruence. In spite of the fact that a unique representation is certainly the ultimate goal, it is unlikely that such a representation can actually be defined and implemented. On the other hand, the different representation schemes (i.e. voxel, surface, oct-tree. etc.) that will be considered useful must, at least, be congruent in the sense that each one must be obtainable from all the others. This will assure a real Integration of the volumetric information.

- Incrementability. It is unlikely that a sophisticated model like the one that we propose to develop can be obtained from a single information source or in a single processing step. It is more likely that the model will be obtained through an iterative procedure controlled by the operator. For this reason the representation schema should be definable incrementally.

- Robustness. The modelling technique (and the representation schema) must not be sensible to noise at all the processing levels.

The processing steps that we intend to investigate are:

- Interactive processing and sectioning
    a) reslicing;
    b) numerical projections;
    c) 3D/4D image editing;

- Display of volumetric data
    a) surface display;
    b) voxel display;
    c) movie generation;

- Interactive Numerical Surgery
    a) pointing to anatomical landmark;
    b) cutting;
    c) erasing;
    d) pulling, squeezing, pushing;
    e) 2D and 3D metric primitives (distance, area, volume etc.).

In the following, particular potential activities related to the Multidimensional Image Modelling area are reported.

3.2.1 Data Quantitative Significance

This activity deals with the important problem to assign physical meaning to the measured data. Therefore, physical and mathematical modelling of the measuring systems and measurement procedures will be carried out, with particular attention to the acquisition phase. The goal of characterizing a given acquisition system (such as, for example, MR, PET or US for the image formation step and the meaning of the acquired image intensity pixel by pixel) will produce the benefit to ensure the user of obtaining repeatable data. This objective will be achieved through the realization of software (and, in some instances, hardware) modules which will be currently applied as "quantitative correcting" filters through simple system calls. More in general, this work will produce improvement in the basic knowledge of each specific technique, eventually allowing its best use in the current clinical practice.

3.2.2 Rigid Objects

This activity will deal with the definition of modelling techniques for human body segments such as bones which can be modelled using information deriving from Xray and MR techniques. Generation procedures can be set up using geometric primitives - when applicable - and norms established on the basis of Xray and MR images available or, when necessary, obtained for this purpose. Processing procedures would include techniques to build up 3D shapes - on the basis of which norms and changes away from norms, specially when particular pathologies are present, can be specified.

3.2.3 Articulated Objects

Human body segments such as multiple body structures require the definition of the same generation, processing and coding procedures as rigid object. A definition phase about information on links among parts of the structure, constraints on movement and relationships among parts of complex structures would be added. As refers to linguistic information, hierarchical knowledge organization would be suitable.

3.2.4 Continuum-like Deformable Objects

Body segments whose shape varies can be modelled using information deriving from Xray, MR, US, PET and nuclear medicine techniques. Functional 3D images (like, for example, images representing blood flow, absorption of particular substances or other functional parameters versus time) can also be regarded as continuum-like deformable objects. With respect to the case of rigid objects, they would require for the generation, processing and coding procedures the implementation of specific algorithms based on approaches such as tensorial calculus or other analytically complex techniques. As object complexity in this case is greater then in the previous cases, linguistic information procedures would be more complex, and, therefore, Artificial Intelligence Techniques such as qualitative reasoning could be an appropriate tool.

References

M. L. Brodic, J. Mylopoulos: *"Knowledge Base Management Systems"*. Springer Verlag. 1986.

D. L. Burk, D. C. Mears, W. H. Kennedy, L. A. Cooperstein, D. L. Herbert: "Three dimensional Computed Tomography of Acetabular Fractures". *Radiology,* 1985; 155: pp183-186.

R. L. Cook: "Shade Trees". *Computer Graphics.* 1984; 18, No. 3: pp. 223-231.

R. L. Cook, L. Carpenter and E. Catmull: "The Reyes Image Rendering Architecture". *Computer Graphics.* 1987; 21, No. 4: pp. 95-102.

F. C. Crow: "A More Flexible Image Generation Environment". *Computer Graphics.* 1982; 16, No.3: pp. 9-18.

T. Duff: "Compositing 3D Rendered Images". *Computer Graphics.* 1985; 19, No. 3: pp. 41-44.

N. Ezquerra, E. Garcia: "Artificial Intelligence gives Computer New Role as Imaging Problem-Solver". *Medical Imaging,* 1985: pp. 195-200.

A. Fagot Largeault: "La Simulation du Raisonnement Medical". *La Recherche*. 1985:pp. 1176-1187.

H. Fuchs, G. D. Abram, E. D. Grant: "Near real-time shaded display of rigid objects". *Computer Graphics*. 1983; 17 No.3: pp 65-72.

W. V. Glenn, R. J. Johnson, P. E. Morton, S. J. Dwyer: "Image generation and Display Techniques for CT scan data". *Investigative Radiology*. 1975; 10 No.5: pp 403-416.

S. M. Goldwasser: "A Generalized Object Display Processor Architecture". *IEEE Computer Graphics and Applications*. 1984; 4 No.10: pp 43-55.

S. M. Goldwasser, D. Reynolds, D. Talton, E. Walsh: "Real time Display and Manipulation of 3-D CT, PET, and NMR data". Int. Workshop on Physics and Engineering in Computerized Multidimensional Imaging and Processing. 1986.

R. A. Hall and D. P. Greenberg: "A Testbed for Realistic Image Synthesis". *IEEE Comp. Graphics and Applications*. 1983; 3 No.11: pp. 10-20.

L. D. Harris, R. A. Robb, T. S. Yuen, E. L. Ritman: "Display and Visualization of three-dimensional reconstructed anatomic morphology: experience with the torax, heart and coronary vasculature of dogs ". *Journal Computer assisted Tomography*. 1979; 3: pp 439-446.

A. W. Paeth and K. S. Booth: "Design and Experience with a Generalized Raster Toolkit". Graphics interface 1986 Proceedings.1986; pp. 91-97.

R. B. Pearce: "Expert Systems enable Computers to share in Imaging Decisions". Medical Imaging. 1947; pp. 146-152.

K. Perlin: "An Image Synthesizer". Computer Graphics. 1985; 19 No. 3: pp. 287-286.

T. Porter and T. Duff: "Compositing Digital Images". *Computer Graphics* . 1984; 18 No. 3: pp. 253-259.

Potmesil M. and Hoffert E.M.: "FRAMES: Software Tools for Modeling, Rendering and Animation of 3D Scenes". *Computer Graphics*. 1987; 21 No. 4: pp. 85-93.

Proceedings of the IEEE, Special Issue on Distributed Database Systems, 1987; 75 n° 5. 1

Tsotsos J.K.: "Computer Assessment of Left Ventricular Wall Motion: the ALVEN Expert System". *Computer & Biomedical Research*. 1985; 18: pp. 254-277.

Whitted T. and Weimer D.M.: "A Software Testbed for the Development of 3D Raster Graphics Systems". *ACM Transactions on Computer Graphics* . 1982; 1 No. 1: pp. 43-58.

Williams T.: "Optics and Neural Nets: Trying to Model the Human Brain". *Computer Design*. 1987; 26 n°5: pp. 47-62.

Herman G.T.: "The Tracking of Boundaries in 3D Medical Images". *Proc 9th Int Conf Pattern Recognition* . 1988; pp. 998-1003.

Hohne K.H., Bomans M., Pommert A., Riemer M. and Tiede U.: "3D-Segmentation and Display of Tomographic Imagery" . *Proc 9th Int Conf Pattern Recognition*. 1988; pp. 1271-1276.

Sequeira J.: "Modèlisation Interactive d'Objets de Forme Complexe à Partir de Données Hétérogènes" . PhD Thesis, Univ Franche Comte. 1987; pp. 1-195.

Terzopoulus D.,Witkin A. and Kass M.: "Constraints on Deformable Models: Recovering 3D Shape and Nonrigid Motion". *Artificial Intelligence*. 1988; 36: pp.91-123.

Kelly P.J., Alker G.J. , Zoll J.G.: "A microstereotaxic approach to deep-seated arteriovenous malformations". *Surg Neurol* . 1982; 17:pp. 260-262.

Kelly P.J., Bruce A.K., Goerss B.S., Earnest F.: "Computer assisted stereotaxic laser resection of intra-axial brain neoplasms". *J Neurosurg* . 1986; 4 n°64: pp.427-439.

Andrew G., Watkins E.S. : "A stereotaxic atlas of the human thalamus and adjacent structures, a variability study ". The Williams & Wilkins Co.

Beltrame F., Rolandelli M.L., Sandini G., Tagliasco V.: "Integration between Information and Optical Media-Based Technologies for Medical Knowledge Transmission". *Journal of Clinical Computing*. 1987; 16, n° 3. 1988 ; 4, pp. 104-131.

Beltrame F.: "Eidologia e Sapere Medico". *Sapere.* 1987; 53, n° 7, pp. 27-32.

Beltrame F., Rolandelli M.L.,Sandini G.,Tagliasco V.: "Integration of Biomedical Images for Medical Knowledge Representation". *Proc. XIVth Congress of the European Society of Neuroradiology*, CIC Edizioni Internazionali. 1987; pp. 583-590 .

P A C S and Radiotherapy

Inger-Lena Lamm* and Torgil Möller#
*Department of Radiation Physics, #Department of Oncology,
University Hospital, S-221 85 Lund, Sweden

1   General introduction

The acronym PACS was introduced in connection with the "First International Conference and Workshop on Picture Archiving and Communication Systems (PACS) for Medical Applications" in 1982 (1). PACS in themselves were no novelties; manual analog PACS were and are abundant. Even today imaging departments still rely heavily on "manual retrieval and transmission" of analog radiographic films from central film rooms, of floppy disks and mag-tape reels containing digital CT-images etc. The novelty was the concept of a "computer-assisted PACS" as the first step towards a filmless medical imaging department, and the systematic approach to the problems of image retrieval, communication and archiving.

Today, definition of a second generation of PACS is appearing (2), "which integrates image generation, display and analysis, storage (both short term and archival), production of hardcopy, communication between all of the subsystems and between systems, and management of both the images and the system." The scope of these second generation systems is thus much wider than that of the first generation, implying integration with other information systems, such as Hospital Information Systems (HIS) and Radiology Information Systems (RIS); not only to support image management but also to integrate the use of image and non-image data (2, 3). To distinguish the latter type of system functionality, new acronymes such as IMACS - Image Management And Communication Systems - have been created (the translation Information Management And Communication Systems fits as well); or why not use MACS - Medical Archiving and Communication Systems - for an integrated information system in medicine?

Developments and tests of PACS have been dedicated mostly to the field of diagnostic radiology, with emphasis on the requirements of the diagnosticians as "human viewers". But, other users of images, e.g. in radiotherapy and surgery, must also specify their needs. In future generalized PACS, image analysis functions are expected to play an increasingly important role.

After a shorter discussion on some aspects of introducing information technology in medicine, some of the specific PACS requirements for radiotherapy are considered, as well as future developments of computer assistance to use "all knowledge available" -computer vision tools - and a futuristic radiotherapist multi-modality workstation.

2   Introduction of information technology in medicine

The introduction of information technology in the clinical environment will always affect the organization of a department; new routines, new tasks, who does what, new distribution of influence etc. New technology often works as a catalyst, bringing organization problems to the fore. Common incentives for introducing new technologies are expected increases in quality and flexibility, decreases of operational costs and more direct control of management. Large effects should not be expected until some time after the introduction of new systems; the users first have to learn to do things correctly, after that they will be ready to start doing the correct things, i.e. exploiting the possibilities of the system and thus pushing new developments.

2.1 Introduction of PACS

PACS is definitely not "just a product, but a way of thinking" (4). The PACS concept covers the whole organization of the "PACS clinic", and the different types of medical workstations with their different functions could be regarded as the "interfaces" between the human users and the PACS. The computer assisted PACS and their subsystems will allow the introduction of completely new tools, which in themselves also will affect the ways of working with images on all application levels.

PACS components exist and are used increasingly in clinical routine, but today dominantly as stand-alone subsystems. To get not only a passive user acceptance but an active user participation, it is imperative that the user community is encouraged to participate from the beginning in defining requirements for the PACS and their subsystems.

The digital images from all imaging modalities should be displayed and evaluated interactively in PACS workstations, which primarily correspond to the conventional lightboxes used for films. These workstations should not only replace the boxes but also give an "added value"; they will, as mentioned, be able to provide new tools for evaluation purposes. But, what are the requirements for the workstations to be accepted in the clinical routine; to make them, in the first place, at least as good as the old lightboxes for the human viewer? And, what are the specific requirements and the added value expected for the specialized workstations used e.g. in radiotherapy? The way humans function must be considered; we are, for instance, very good at "comparing" images when we see them side by side but definitely not if we have to remember one or several of them. These latter aspects belong to the field of human-computer-interfaces (HCI), and the definition and design of the HCI is a challenge in itself. Refereses on different aspects of computer assisted radiology can be found in (5).

3   The radiotherapy information system today

In order to find the "optimal" way of delivering radiotherapy to an individual patient, we must use all knowledge available; i.e. knowledge about host factors and tumour factors for the specific patient as well as knowledge about patients treated earlier, given as both image and non-image information. In an integrated radio-therapy information system, fulfilling the clinical requirements, all relevant data should be available at the different steps in the radiotherapy procedure. The system should also include appropriate tools for handling these image and non-image data.

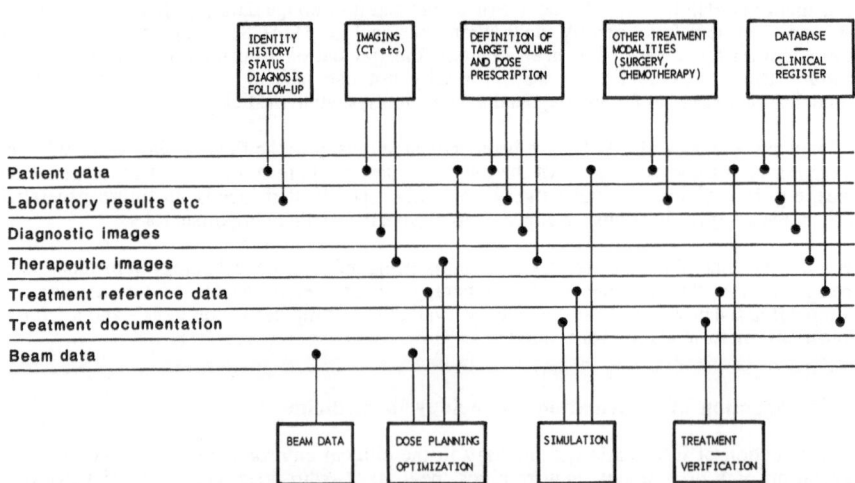

Representation of the flow of information within a radiotherapy department. The different types of data are represented as horizontal logical network channels, the boxes represent the steps of the radiotherapy procedure, and each dot marks information exchange as input and/or output to the network. The data flow in the two image channels is vastly greater than in the other channels. IMAGING stands for all types of image acquisition. (Reproduced from ICRU 42 (6).).

Thus, such a system belongs to the class of second generation PACS, and is schematically illustrated above.

3.1 Images in radiotherapy - PACS aspects

Traditionally, images are used abundantly in radiotherapy procedures:
o   in treatment planning to define tumour and target volumes and to define the optimal irradiation technique for the patient
o   in treatment delivery to verify the equivalence between planned and given treatment;
o   in follow-up to evaluate and record treatment response.

Modern treatment planning should be based on
o   a description of the patient in 3D (4D when time is included) geometrically: tumour and target volumes, organs at risk.physically: relative electron densities...
o   a description of the treatment units (sources) in 3D (4D)
o   a model for calculating biological treatment effects in the patient (absorbed dose in space-time, in the future including the effect of other treatment modalities as well)

Tools should be available to
o   integrate all types of image information in 3D, projections as well as sections (CT, MRI, US etc..)
o   handle/analyze/present patient information, image (in 3D-4D) and non-image
o   define treatment beams and sources in relation to the patient in 3D
o   evaluate/optimize intended/given radiotherapy: present "patient + treatment + effect" in 3D
o   verify given treatment
o   perform Quality Assurance of the treatment procedure

In radiotherapy, as well as in some surgical specialties, exact 3D information about the patient is crucial. Hence the potential of volumetric imaging was first acknowledged in those disciplines. References on Computers in Radiotherapy can be found in (7).

Computers have been used for decades now in radiotherapy for "dose planning"; they and their display terminals, "workstations" as it were, are no strangers. The early dose planning "workstations" were simple compared to the requirements above, which are part of the specifications for a dedicated radiotherapy workstation, RTWS, capable of interactive image handling and treatment modelling. Some of the specific PACS aspects of these workstations are considered below.

Concerning selective retrieval and response time in using images, the RTWS must allow interactive access to all the images for the active patient during planning, i.e. instantaneous (<1-2 sec) display of whatever image is asked for. The emphasis in RT on 3D presentation and image integration is strong. The RT procedure of today makes it possible to use some simple type of prefetching of image data for the active patients, both from central archives and from local image sources such as a dedicated radiotherapy CT-scanner and a conventional simulator. The prefetching of patient data could be initiated well in advance of a planning session, and performed during non-busy periods. Thus, neither response time nor selective retrieval are problems for this application, as long as the active images can be temporarily stored locally in an interactive RTWS.

A way of enhancing the response time of a system, as well as reducing storage requirements, is to use data compression techniques. The method of compression must be related to the purpose of doing it (8); lossy irreversible compression might be used when the purpose is simply to view the image. Suffice it here to state that only the reversible compression techniques, preserving the image content, are at present acceptable for quantitative use of the data and when image processing is to be performed. From the radiotherapist's point of view it is further to be noted that a data reduction, where specific images are selected entirely from a diagnostic point of view, is not acceptable; a full 3D representation of the patient requires not only e.g. the CT slices where the tumour is shown, but also images (information) covering the
total volume to be irradiated.

Storage of RT-images should be distributed to the RT-department. The RTWS allows the user to pick anatomical images - either as "raw unprocessed images" or with some markings from processing e.g. in the diagnostic department, and produces a patient representation consisting of organs, target volume etc, a density volume for dose distribution calculations, a beam/source representation, a treatment effect volume and various computer generated images. The RT images are of interest primarily in the RT department and should be used extensively for treatment verification, quality assurance of the treatment procedure and for follow-up studies.

The image analysis/processing part of the RTWS is in its infancy, and will be considered briefly in section 4.

To summarize the present status, we have today the basic tools to "handle" 3D image information, but we do not have the tools available to really help in managing all the information and extracting the relevent parts of it in an intelligent way.

4   Future Developments of the integrated radiotherapy information system

In a future PACS system, the user will be able to pick up information at different workstations. These workstations should be "identical", i.e. they should present the same types of information in the same way, and the tools should be recognized as performing specific functions in the same way. It is further essential that the user gets confirmation from the system that the correct information has been used, be it image or non-image. The tools should ideally help the user to use his/her own competence in a better way. To design the tools required in radiotherapy, several of which might be common to other clinical disciplines and already available, we must have an extensive model of the radiotherapy procedure, remembering that radiotherapy is one of the several cancer treatment modalities.

The management of a patient could be described schematically in three steps: i) definition of the specific treatment (based on cancer care programs); ii) planning and delivery of treatment (according to the program); iii) evaluation and follow-up (results achieved according to predefined endpoints in the program).We will here concentrate on the development of tools to help the user handle the image information.

4.1 Computer Vision in radiotherapy
The tools required to plan, verify and evaluate radiotherapy treatments have been presented in section 3. Experience has shown, that the manual definition of organs and target volume in 3D is atime consuming process. Existing simple semi-automatic methods still leave a lot of the work to the user. The definition of target volume is the crucial step in radiotherapy; the optimal definition of the boundaries of the target volume is that the probability of deposits of tumour cells outside the target volume in curative treatment should approach zero. In the future, tools using computer vision (CV) methods to extract relevant information from images might be the solution to this problem.

Computer vision is a fairly new discipline, combining digital image processing, image analysis, image understanding, neurophysiology, cognitive psychology etc., and it is one of the most challenging areas of artificial intelligence. Experimental systems have already shown the feasibility of using CV methods in clinical radiology (5,9). The radiotherapy applications are in their infancy, but developments towards CV applications have started.

Computer vision is "the construction of explicit meaningful descriptions of physical objects from images" (Ballard, Brown). For our applications, problem areas of interest are: i) How do humansfunction as observers? ii) How do humans reason about images? iii) What is a "visually competent expert system" for treatment planning? iv) What are the clinical requirements? v) How should properties of the objects be described and represented? A project, Computer vision in radiotherapy, has been suggested as one of the continuation projects of the Nordic co-operation programme CART - Computer Aided RadioTherapy (10). The primary aim should be to define user requirements from the clinical experts' points of view and also to evaluate today existing 2D image analysis/processing methods for future 3D applications.

The further aim of the project would be to build a prototype image understanding knowledgebased system for radiotherapy, consisting of three modules with the following tasks:

o to build a 3D model of the patient based on a general geometric representation of reference man/woman
o to suggest reference target volumes in the patient based on tumour site and stage according to specific cancer care programs
o to suggest treatment techniques based on target volume, specified dose levels and reference techniques according to cancer care programs.

The computer vision tasks to be addressed are as follows:

o define reference man/woman - organs and anatomical landmarks
o define compartments in reference man/woman
o define reference target volumes in relation to tumour site and stage in reference man/woman
o recognize organs and anatomical landmarks in patient
o define a mapping from reference man/woman to patient
o define compartments in patient and suggest target volumes
o compare several examinations with different time intervals to
     - study variation in tumour volume
     - calculate remission grade
     - verify local control
     - define recurrence in relation to original target volume and dose distribution (failure analysis)
     - study nonlinear changes in irradiated tissue volume.

The development of image understanding procedures is important in many other areas, such as image-key retrieval from image databases and use of symbolic image descriptions for specialized knowledge-based systems. Medical images are difficult, and we are definitely some way from a system "that can automatically produce a good symbolic representation of the shape of a nonrigid, poorly defined structure in the presence of other structures", as stated in (11).

4.2 The radiotherapist workstation
We have been playing with a vision of a futuristic radiotherapist workstation, in terms of functional user requirements. This work-station should not only replace the piles of patient records, forms to be filled in etc, but in addition truly support the user in the daily routine.

With the radiotherapist workstation, it should be quick and easy to fetch images (perhaps provided with "spoken" comments) for viewing purposes, and to compare images e.g. to see if a tumour is changing in size. The traditional patient record should be available simultaneously; for quick perusal - humans are very good at flipping through pages to find the relevant piece of information - and for thorough reading. Retrieval of similar cases should be possible, with "similar" defined by the user. Laboratory test should be presented as graphs if desired, e.g. with the requested test values given as functions of time. Standard template images (in 3D) should be available, where the therapist could draw a tumour and get a suggestion for TNM classification. Knowledgebased support systems should help in managing treatments, determining therapy, suggesting preliminary reference irradiation techniques etc, and also in presenting pertinent reference literature. Further, it would be of great importance also for educational purposes to have both reference cases and a library readily available. Scribbles should be made on a memo pad and also directly on images, and the user should be able to interact by pointing at "things" and by using his/her voice. The workstation "should behave as expected", and be very forgiving towards user abuse and misbehaviour. It should further be possible to use ordinary analog paper as well while working, requiring a horisontal surface of at least part of the workstation.

PACS (or IMACS) is the necessary invisible giant behind this formidable multi modality workstation, integrating information, handling archives, communications, retrievals, data security etc. Such a workstation would be used not only by radiotherapists, but by all oncologists and many other specialists as well, after suitable adaptions.

References:

1) A.J. Duerinckx: (ed.) Proc of the First Int. Conf. on Picture Archiving and Communication (PACS) for Medical Applications. *Proc. SPIE* 1982: 318

2) G.Q. Maguire, M.E.Noz, A. Bakker, K. Bijl, H. Didden and J.P.J. de Valk.: Introduction to PACS for Those Interested in Image Processing (IPMI 1987) *Information Processing in Medical Imaging*, De Graaf C.N. and Viergever M.A. (eds), Plenum Press, New York, in press

3) J.P.J. de Valk, A.R. Bakker, K. Bijl, W. Heijser, D.E. Boekee and G.L. Reijns: PACS Reviewed: Possible and Coming Soon? MEDINFO 86, R. Salamon, B. Blum and M. Jorgensen (Eds), Elsevier Science Publishers B.V. (North-Holland)

4) D. Meyer-Ebrecht: The PACS concept- not a product, but a way of thinking. New Imaging 1988:1

5) Computer Assisted Radiology, CAR'85 and CAR'87. H.U. Lemke et al (eds), Springer-Verlag, Berlin, 1985, 1987

6) Use of Computers in External Beam Radiotherapy Procedures with High-Energy Photons and Electrons.ICRU Report 42 (International Commmission on Radiation Units and Measurements), Bethesda, Maryland, 1987

7) The Use of Computers in Radiation Therapy, I.A.D. Bruinvis et al (eds), Elsevier Science Publishers B.V. (North-Holland), 1987

8) A. Todd-Pokropek: Image data compression techniques: a survey. In: Mathematics and Computer Science in Medical Imaging, M.A. Viergever and A. Todd-Pokropek (eds), NATO ASI Series F:39, Springer-Verlag, Berlin, 1988

9) H.S. Stiehl:. On Spatial Image Sequence Understanding. Habilitation Monograph. Technische UniversitÑt Berlin, 1987

10) I.-L. Lamm. CART - report on the Nordic co-operation programme. Journal of Medical Imaging, 2 (1988) 44-49

11) J Fox and N. Walker: Knowledge based interpretation of medical images. Mathematics and Computer Science in Medical Imaging, M.A. Viergever and A. Todd-Pokropek (eds), NATO ASI Series F:39, Springer-Verlag, Berlin, 1988

Advanced Medical Robotics

by Patrick A. Finlay and Paul D. Wilson
Fulmer Systems Ltd., United Kingdom

One of the most striking things about medical robots is how few of them there are. Another is the large number of research projects internationally aimed at getting medical robots into service as early as possible. What is it that has suddenly happened to make robots good news for patients and doctors? And what sort of jobs will medical robots be able to tackle?

To answer the second question first, the scope for robots in health care is vast. Three general categories of task can be distinguished: rehabilitation functions, aimed at restoring mobility to the disabled; hospital service functions covering materials handling tasks in hospitals and clinical functions, involving direct interaction with patients A recent series of brainstorm sessions between physicians and robot engineers, organised by Fulmer Research in the United Kingdom, identified over 400 possible applications ranging from intelligent artificial limbs to microsurgery. Three of these ideas are now the subject of development programmes under the UK Advanced Robotics initiative.

It is not difficult to understand why medical robots have been so long in coming. One reason is product liability. Industrial robots are normally required to be fenced to the full extent of their working envelope to prevent accidents to people. Medical robots, almost by definition, are designed to interact physically with people, often in intimate procedures such as teeth brushing for the disabled or brain tumour surgery (to name two current examples). Furthermore, the people concerned are frequently unable to activate an emergency stop if a malfunction occurs. It's only with the development of 3rd generation robots with sophisticated sensor systems and substantial real-time processing power that such human/robot interaction can be contemplated. Earlier experimenters in medical robotics were obliged to downgrade their system performance in terms of torque and speed in order to reduce risks, but the resultant specification was unacceptably poor.

Another brake on the development of health care automation generally has been the well-known culture gap between physicians and engineers. In the medical profession, new equipment is introduced by persuading a well respected consultant to conduct clinical trials and write an approving commendation. Unfortunately consultants have nothing to gain from conducting clinical trials, but ·a lot to lose in terms of reputation if the trials go wrong. They are therefore understandably conservative in their approach to new ideas unless they have been closely involved with a project from its start.

A further disincentive for robots in medicine has been a psychological aversion on the part of patients and their carers about being dealt with by an automaton rather than a human. A robot would not have the compassion and understanding of a nurse, whilst the prospect of robot surgery is even less conducive to patient well-being than the human variety. The answer to these points, of course, is that there is no suggestion of nurses or surgeons being replaced by robots, but there is a good case for providing these professionals with intelligent tools to enable them to do their jobs better. In the UK, 750,000 nursing days are lost each year due to back injuries, mostly caused by lifting bedridden patients. An intelligent lifting device would save that waste and release nurses to do the job for which they are trained. It would also give the patient the dignity of, for example, going to the bath alone rather than with enforced company.

Much the same fears of dehumanisation were associated with industrial robots during the early 1970's, but once robots had been installed in a factory it amazed the sceptics how rapidly the management and workforce accepted them as just another piece of plant. Doubtless the same will happen in healthcare.

The drive for robots in medicine has taken a new impetus with the realisation that all developed countries have greying populations. 18% of the UK population is currently aged 65 or over, and the percentage is growing. The consequent increased demand for healthcare services is made more serious by the fall in the number of people of working age. Automation in healthcare has been recommended by WHO (the World Health Organisation) as a priority for developed countries. Add to this the fact that the current generation of physicians and paramedics has grown up with computer-based medical equipment, such as digital imaging systems and therefore does not suffer from techno-fear, and the fact that patients themselves are more kindly disposed toward a high-tech hospital environment ; and it becomes clear that the opportunities for advanced robotics in medicine and healthcare are considerable.

But they do have to be advanced robot systems - third generation robotics which include real time interactive sensor feedback, expert system and IKB system intelligence; capable of at least semi-autonomous operation, including mobility and navigation where necessary. They will also require user interfaces which break new ground in the fields of ergonomics and MMI/HCI. A key feature of these robots will be their ability to interpret unstructured situations and make decisions based on less-than-perfect informations. In order to improve the quality of these decisions, it is clearly important to present the robot with all the available information, structured in such a way that easy assimilation of vital data is possible. In the context of surgical robotics, the information which is most useful in itentifying features and performing diagnosis is nearly all in the form of digital medical images, obtained from a wide variety of imaging modelities.That is why the link between PACS and surgery robotics is so strong, for PACS provides sensor data in a format which can be readily interrogated by the robot cell computer, both pre-operatively in planning an intervention and in real time (if suitable preparations are made) whilst a procedure is in progress.

Systems such as this do not currently exist, but they are not far from the market place. In the field of rehabilitation, for example, the Japanese "Meldog" guide robot for the blind is undergoing pre-production trials.This powered mobile trolley is able to navigate around a town using a pre-stored map in its memory. On-board sensors are used to identify street junctions based on the disposition of walls and signposts. Other sensors detect obstructions and navigate around them. Meldog communicates with its blind owner via a radio link to a special belt which generates a mild electric stimulus warning the wearer to stop, or to prepare to turn left or right. Meldog itself senses the owner's walking speed, and remains a metre or two ahead.

Another development from Japan is the "Transfer Supporting System for the Handicapped" - an AGV system for transporting bedridden patients between various locations in a hospital. Each AGV carries a patient transfer device consisting of a board with contra-rotating belts above and below.This can be driven between the patient and his mattress without relative sliding, enabling the patient then to be translated to the AGV itself for transport. The board is hinged in two places, enabling it to be configured as a seat during the transport phase.

Undoubtedly the application area offering the most exciting prospects is that of the clinical use of robots for diagnosis, therapy and surgery. There are a number of surgical procedures which are currently limited by the accuracy achievable by a surgeon. For example in opthalmic micro-surgery, a radial keratotomy procedure ideally requires a depth of cut in the cornea controlled to 20 microns. A good surgeon can manage 100 microns, which is impressive, but a robot currently under development in Canada will be able to match the ideal figure. Other examples where high precision is required are found in microneurosurgery. A Puma robot in the US has been demonstrated extracting brain tumour tissue for biopsy, using the result of a stereotactic scan to plan the optimum trajectory for its drill, which is only 2 mm diameter. Another development is underway in France to use a robot to assist in a spinal repair procedure, where an error could result in paralysis of the patient. Again, in Japan, a robot has been demonstrated in a corneal transplant procedure (not on a live patient).

As well as precision, another advantage of robots is their ability to undertake complex sequences of movements. In the UK, a robot has been demonstrated by a team from Imperial College and the Institute of Urology in a simulated prostate surgery operation. Prostate surgery involves an intricate pattern of cuts and it is difficult for human surgeons to keep track of where they are in the sequence.

A further field of clinical interest is the use of robots to reduce the dangers of biological or other hazards. Radiotherapy is an obvious prospect here, particularly the use of a single robot to replace many expensive stationary sources in multi-beam targeted radiotherapy. A European development of a radiotherapy manipulator is at an early stage. A number of existing medical imaging devices, such as CT (computer assisted tomography) scanners already use robotic principles for manipulating patients, and this can be expected to spread.

All this interest and activity indicates that computer assisted intervention is about to make a significant impact into clinical practice. It is true to say that at the moment everyone's experience is still at the lower end of the learning curve, but once the enabling technologies are developed, it will not be long before surgical robots are assisting human surgeons to carry out procedures which are currently considered inoperable, improving the prognosis for patients across a wide spectrum of clinical classification.

Professor Mike Brady of Oxford University has defined robotics as "the intelligent connection of perception to action". In the context of surgery robotics, the difficulty of the task requires more than the normal level of machine intelligence and perception. The link between PACS, as an intelligent information gathering and communication system, and robotics, which interprets sensor information into action, is clear. The two technologies are complementary, and it is vital that an aspect of future PACS developments should be the creation of effective interfaces between intelligent surgery manipulators, human surgeons and medical images. Medical robotics is undoubtedly a key tool of the operating theatre of the future.

The importance of the field was recognised in 1982 when the heads of state ang governments of the DECD established the International Advanced Robotics Programme as part of the Versailles summit meeting. Medical applications was one of the 10 areas specifically targeted by the programme, and the United Kingdom was chosen to be the lead country in this area, with Japan, the USA and Canada as collaborators. Within the UK, the department of Trade and Industry appointed Fulmer Research, a private contract research and technology organisation, to carry out an initial feasibility study to identify suitable application areas for development. The Fulmer team, assisted by medical, robot ad AI specialists from UK industry and universities, identified three targets: a surgery assistant robot, a patient handling robot and a fetch and carry robot for the disabled. Clubs of industrial and academic collaborators have been established to embark on parallel 3-year programmes to develop demonstrator systems incorporating 3rd generation robot technology. Unlike existing research programmes wich are directed towards solving specific problems, these projects are directed towards developing the generic enabling technologies necessary for advanced medical robots. In surgery,these include tissue discrimination, the surgeon/robot interface, patient calibration, computer modelling of the human body, and medical imaging data compression and fusion. the last of these is also the province of PACS, and stresses the need for close co-operation between PACS experts and medical robot engineers.

Medical robot is thus in a particularly exciting position: current application examples are few and their technology is behind that of industrial robots, but research labs around the world are developing advanced products which will revolutionise whole areas of health care. The market is a rapidly growing one, and Europe is well placed to be a leader, due to a unique combination of expertise in both robotic research, medical automation applications and PACS developments. If Europe seizes the opportunity to interface PACS and medical robotics, there is every opportunity for us to lead the world in this exciting and rapidly growing field.

Advanced Interfaces for Teleoperated Robotic Surgery

P. Dario, M. Bergamasco, A. Sabatini
Scuola Superiore S. Anna, Pisa
Centro "E. Piaggio", University of Pisa, Italy

The control of a multifingered hand slave in order to accurately exert arbitrary forces and impart small movements to a grasped object, such as a surgery tool, is a knotty problem in robotic teleoperation, and, more specifically, in teleoperated surgery.

Although a number of articulated robotic hands have been proposed in the recent past for dexterous manipulation in autonomous robots, the possible use of such hands as slaves in teleoperated manipulation and surgery is hindered by the present lack of sensors in those hands, and (even if those sensors were available) by the inherent difficulty of transmitting to the master operator the complex sensations elicited by such sensors at the slave level.

In this paper an analysis of different problems related to sensor-based telemanipulation is presented. The general sensory systems requirements for dexterous slave manipulators are pointed out and the description of a practical sensory system set-up for the robotic system we have developed is presented.

The problem of feeding-back to the human master operator stimuli that can be interpreted by his central nervous system as originated during real dexterous manipulation and surgery is then considered. Examples of devices usable as man-machine interfaces for controlling fine teleoperated surgical operations are given. Finally, some preliminary work aimed at developing an advanced man-machine interface consisting of an instrumented glove incorporating Kevlar tendons and tension sensors is described. The interface is designed purposely for navigating into 3D body representations incorporating models of tissue mechanics, and for controlling teleoperated microsurgery.

1 Introduction

Teleoperated robots can be particularly useful in many surgical tasks, and especially in microsurgery, where they can significantly enhance the performance of the surgeon. Telemanipulation, a fundamental task in robotic surgery, requires high dexterity and complex sensorymotor control procedures. Furthermore, being ultimately aimed at extending the sensing and manipulation capabilities of the human operator to the slave robotic system, telemanipulation requires not only a dexterous slave end-effector, but also a sensory system able to sense and transmit complex tactile and kinestetic sensations.

A number of articulated robotic hands have been proposed in the recent past in the field of autonomous robotics for dexterous manipulation (1) (2). The use of such hands as "slaves" in teleoperated manipulation and surgery is hindered primarily by the present lack of sensors in those hands. Furthermore, even if those sensors were available, it would be inherently difficult to convey to the surgeon the complex sensations elicited by such sensors at the slave level. This is a fundamental problem in telesurgery: the telemanipulation system should allow the surgeon not only to observe the manipulated body part, but even to feel the physical contact with it.

Current state of the art in telemanipulated end-effectors includes joysticks and handles, or grippers, incorporating some simple sensors. At the master device level, some additional sophistication has been achieved with the DataGlove (3), which incorporates fiberoptic position sensors located at the finger joints, and a 6-degree-of-freedom tracking device mounted at the wrist which provides information about position, orientation and whole configuration of the human operator hand in 3D space.

It is the objective of the research activity we are carrying out in our laboratory to investigate the design principles and to identify the main problems involved in the development of a master-slave system which could be used for sensor-based telemicromanipulation and surgery. In particular our ultimate goal is to render a surgeon able to control a multifingered hand slave in a truly dexterous way, that is to accurately exert arbitrary forces and impart small movements to a surgical tool located in a remote operational space.

In the following some basic considerations on the design of a telemanipulation system are discussed first. These considerations are related to the general system architecture and to the requirements for slave and master devices, as well as to the sensory systems which have to be integrated in their structures in order to achieve an active bilateral control of the manipulative operation. The following paragraphs deal with the description of a simple robotic system we are currently developing in order to investigate some basic issues in telemicromanipulation for robotic surgery. The robotic system consists of a tendon actuated robotic slave finger with joint rotation and torque sensors and tactile sensors at the fingertip, and of an anthropomorphic glove-like exoskeleton incorporating actively controlled joints for reproducing kinesthetic sensations on the master human operator (4).

2 General design considerations for a robotic system for teleoperated surgery

As a first step towards the development of a telemanipulation system for robot surgery, we have attempted to define some general specifications both on the principles of operation (for example, the way in which the whole process could be performed) and on the specific hardware characteristics that a master-slave system should possess for carrying out telemicromanipulated surgical procedures.

As far as the human control of the remote surgical task is concerned, we assume that the surgeon will usually not just supervise the operation and leave the responsibility of executing semi-automated manipulation procedures to the robotic system. As we assume a direct and continuous human control on the operation, we have conceived a strict isomorphic relation (*isomorphism*) between the robotic hand and the human master hand.

The isomorphic assumption leads to a clear emphasis in our approach for the concept of telepresence (or tele-existence) of which the telemanipulation task represents only one (although fundamental, because it is "active") aspect. For this reason, we have imagined a scenario conceptually rather similar to that already introduced in the virtual display-control interface for the DataGlove (4), where the surgeon, wearing a video display in which the video image of the operational space is represented, feels himself as present in the remote working place. It is worth observing that this approach is valid not only for executing surgical operations, but also for planning and simulating interventions. In this case the operator could "navigate" inside a computer representation of the human body: most realistic sensations could be transmitted to the remote operator provided that the representation includes a model of the mechanical properties of body tissues.

In analogy with the expected performance of the visual feedback in the case of ideal telepresence, we assume that also the systems designed for feeding-back the contact information detected by the slave robotic hand during manipulation procedures will generate *adequate stimuli* (5) in the human operator hand. The term "adequate stimuli" means that the sensations evoked to the human brain cortex when the manipulation procedure is performed directly by the human hand should be similar to those evoked in the "artificial" situation in which the manipulated surgical procedure is actually performed by the artificial slave hand. This fact implies, that the contact information (i.e. that related to exteroceptors) should be conveied physically to the hand of the surgeon, without any display interface, such as a computer-graphic display or other equivalent devices.

Another important consideration for the definition of a robotic system for telesurgery refers to the availability of a dexterous robotic hand equipped with sensory systems of various kinds. This requirement originates from the very concept of dexterous manipulation, which requires an articulated effector equipped with proprio- and exteroceptive sensors, commanded through a hierarchy of sensory-motor control procedures. In particular, only through an appropriate set of sensors mounted on an artificial dexterous hand the slave will be able to perform "blind" (e.g. without direct visual feedback) tele-commanded operations, a feature that can be useful in cases where vision is impaired, for instance for catheter-based intervention.

From a design point of view, it is important to note that the kinematics of the slave device could even be different from the master's one. The control of the slave in this case would be performed by introducing coordinate transformations. In the particular case the human control is obtained by using an instrumented glove, also the actuation system could be somewhat different from the slave actuation system: in this case a transformation between the master actuator space and the slave actuator space is needed.

3 Sensory requirements for a dexterous slave system

As discussed above, a primary need for a telemanipulation system is the presence of sensory systems located at the slave hand, and capable of extracting information about the contact conditions with the surrounding environment, and in particular with body tissues. These sensory systems, which allow the slave to be controlled during the execution of the complex manipulation procedures required for surgery, can be classified, according to the functional content of the information they extract, as:

a) *teleceptors,* which provide information about the remote operational siteplace as a whole (artificial eyes and ears for long range action; proximity sensors for short range action, etc.);

b) *exteroceptors,* which detect information on the contact between the robot effector and the operational environment (this category includes all the "skin" sensors);

c) *proprioceptors,* which sense position, orientation and relative movements of the various links of the robot effectors (angular joint rotation and internal force sensors);

d) *enteroceptors,* which monitor the functional conditions of the various mechanical and electronic components of the slave system.

All these sensors are essential for the actual control of the whole telemanipulated surgical procedure, as is easy to recognize by considering, for example, how fundamental is the skilled integration of visual and tactile/force sensing modalities for executing even simple manipulation procedures.

We intend to focus our attention on categories b) and c) because these receptors are directly related to the hardware of the slave end-effector .

Contact sensors (external force sensors and tactile sensors) play a very important role, among exteroceptors, on the slave hand. The ability to resolve the six components of the resultant forces and torques acting on the contact regions of the slave hand leads to a more accurate control of manipulative and surgical procedures (6). Force/torque resultant sensors can be positioned either at the wrist of the robotic hand or/and inside the distal phalanxes of each finger, being resolution improved while the sensor moves towards the fingertip. Besides determining contact force and torque, external force/torque resultant sensors provide also extremely useful information about the possible slippage of the surgical tool.

Tactile sensing can be considered as complementary to force sensing for the control of manipulation procedures. Although tactile sensing has been regarded so far in the field of robotics mostly as the artificial sensing modality devoted to determine pressure distribution over the contact regions of the end-effector, "tactile" sensing can actually provide a much wider and larger amount of information. Several technologies have been used to implement the former approach (6). At present, however, not only mechanical but also physical and chemical properties of the contact regions are considered as important and useful for perceptual purposes and for fine manipulation. Real dexterous behavior can result from a synthesis of force and tactile sensing. In fact external force measurements can be effectively combined with the detection of local features, such as the mechanical properties of body tissues in order to more accurately control fine motion and force at the articulated slave hand, thus enhancing the precision of the surgical intervention.

Proprioceptive sensors have the function of indicating to the controller the relative position between the links of the slave hand. The knowledge, at any time, of the "joint vector" allows not only to implement pure position control procedure but also, in combination with internal force/torque information, the hybrid control of manipulation procedures.

In order to demonstrate the importance of providing a slave hand with an appropriate set of exteroceptive and proprioceptive sensory systems, we have implemented a set of simple exploratory procedures by utilizing a tendon actuated, anthropomorphic 4 degree-of-freedom finger equipped with joint rotation and torque internal sensors. The fingertip of the robotic slave is equipped with a multielement tactile sensor (7). We have demonstrated that, by appropriately combining the information provided by the joint position and torque sensors, with that provided by the tactile sensors, it is possible to extract detailed information on body features (e. g. arterial pulse waveform, presence, location, size and depth of nodules embedded in the tissue) through body palpation (8).

4 Considerations on exteroceptive and proprioceptive feedback for a master hand.

Based on the assumption discussed in paragraph 2 of the isomorphic relation between the dexterous robotic slave hand and the human master hand, the problem of specifying the characteristics of the interfacing system has to be addressed. The functional operations required to this interface system are : a) to collect proprioceptive data from the master hand in order to command the slave operation , and b) to transduce the exteroceptive information deriving from the slave into adequate feedback stimuli for the surgeon hand.

Functions a) and b) must be performed by sensory and actuating systems positioned in intimate contact with the hand of the operator, for instance through a deformable or rigid support wrapping the hand up. A clear example of such a structure is the already mentioned DataGlove (3), which incorporates joint angular rotation sensors and allows the hand to reach all possible kinematics configurations.

Manoeuvrability and ergonomic considerations are critical aspects in the design of the master system: these requirements are considerably emphasized in the case of telemicrosurgery, where fine motion control is fundamental. For these reasons it is unlikely that the whole human master system could significantly differ morphologically and functionally from the human hand.

The system we are presently considering for the master surgeon hand consists of an instrumented glove possessing not only position sensors but also an actuating slave-commanded system for finger joints. Kevlar tendons are routed along the back and the palm of the glove in order to actuate directly each phalanx according to a push-pull configuration. Tendon tension sensors, located at the wrist level, control the force-reflecting master-slave and slave-back-to-master procedures. Motors are also located remotely, in a structure beyond the wrist, in order to allow better hand manoeuvrability. An external glove protects the instrumented one and Kevlar transmission tendons. Work is in progress for the realization of a prototype of the tendon-commanded glove.

An open problem for the realisation of a compact and compliant glove-like master device is the definition of the "actuating" or "stimulating" systems aimed at re-creating appropriate exteroceptive stimuli on the virtual contact regions of the human hand. A possible solution to this problem could be the use of local micro-actuators arrays capable of stimulating the human master's hand skin, according to a coherent spatio-temporal pattern. In this context, we are considering some exotic technologies for microactuation, such as solenoid arrays, piezoelectric arrays or micromachined silicon active structures. Even feedback-to-master procedures for replicating "thermal" sensations could be implemented by available technology, should the dimensional vs. manoeuvrability problem find a practical solution.

5 Conclusion

In this paper the general problem of telemanipulation for robotic surgery has been considered. Emphasis has been placed on the particular case of microsurgical tasks, a domain of application that, although extremely challenging for present robot technology, is probably crucial to any wide diffusion of robotics in medicine. We have also mentioned the potential impact on the quality of medical education and training, and on the planning of telesurgical operations, of advanced interfaces which would allow the operator to navigate into computer representations of the patient body   (representations which could be rendered more faithful by appropriately processing real tomographic images, and even data obtained by palpating the patient's body through sensorized robotic probes), and realistically "feel" sensations related to body anatomy.

The simple grippers of ordinary robots will most probably not be sufficient for teleoperated surgery and microsurgery, but even a multifingered robot hand will not be entirely useful if not equipped with adequate sensors. For this reason, the use of joystick-like control devices at the master level will not be entirely satisfactory. An important aspect that we pointed out is that, although the use of joint rotation and torque sensors and of some contact sensors is an essential requirement for dexterous behavior, very fine manipulation requires, in addition, the use of true tactile sensors capable of discriminating fine local details at the finger surface. For microsurgical operations the control of slippage will also be crucial; to this aim, perhaps even a sensitive force/torque fingertip sensor will not suffice, and skin-like distributed tactile sensors capable of sensing locally shear stress will be necessary.

Another important aspect of teleoperation, which to some extent comprises the same functional aspects of the problem, is tele-existence. In this field, sensing the tiny features of contact becomes a key part of the process of perceiving fully a remote reality. Measuring local indentation, and perceiving texture, thermal properties, compliance and other parameters of the touched object by dynamic exploration is a fundamental component of the process by which the surgeon can remotely "construct" a mental image of the surgical field which closely resembles the real one.

Based on the above considerations, we feel that it is extremely important to "enrich" telesensations with information other than just vision. Teletactile sensing is a fundamental (even if not the only) part of the sensory information necessary to the master in order to "generate" a replica of the remote environment as faithful as possible. In this context, particular attention must be devoted to investigate issues of psychophysics, inherently associated with telesensation.

References

1) Salisbury K.: "Teleoperator Hand Design Issues". Proc. of IEEE Intern. Conf. on Robotics and Automation, San Francisco, CA. 1986.

2) Jacobsen S.E. et al. :"The Utah/MIT Dextrous Hand: Work in Progress". *The Int. J. Robotics Res.*. 1984; 3, No. 4.

3) Fisher S. :"Telepresence master glove controller for dexterous robotic end-effectors". *SPIE* Intelligent Robots and Computer Vision: Fifth in a Series, 1986; 726.

4) Andrenucci M., Bergamasco M., Dario P.: "Sensor-based fine telemanipulation for space robotics". Proc. of NASA Conference on Space Telerobotics, Pasadena, CA. January 31-February 2, 1989.

5) Schmidt R.F.:"Fundamentals of Neurophysiology". Springer-Verlag. New York Inc., 1978.

6) Dario P., Bergamasco M., Fiorillo A.S. :"Force and Tactile Sensing for Advanced Robots" in *Sensors and Sensory Systems for Advanced Robots*, Dario P. (Ed.), Springer Verlag, Berlin. 1988.

7) Dario P., Buttazzo G.:"An anthropomorphic robotic finger for investigating artificial tactile perception". *Int. J. Robotics Research*. 1987; 6.

8) Dario P., Bergamasco M.: "An advanced robot system for automated diagnostic tasks through palpation". *IEEE Trans. Biom. Engin.*, 1988;35, No. 2, pp. 118-126.

ISCAMI, PACS & IHIS

D. Pagonis, D. Lacombe*, J. Vermont, F. Berthommier, A. Chapel,
S. Lavallée, I. Marque, P. Cinquin & J. Demongeot
TIMB-TIM3-IMAG, Faculty of Medicine, 38 700 La Tronche, France
* DEC Company, 2 Bd du 11 Novembre, 69626 Villeurbanne Cédex, France

We want to justify in this paper the necessity to build a functionally extensive workstation at the interface between a PACS (Picture Archiving and Communication System) and an IHIS (Integrated Hospital Information System). Such a station will be called an ISCAMI workstation (Integrated System for Computer Assisted Management and Manipulation of Medical Images) and will become one of the main future tools for radiologists, surgeons and clinicians.

1 Building an IHIS

The main aim of an Integrated Hospital Information System (IHIS) is to give an harmonious tool to the clinicians and managers in order to create, send, manipulate and store in a coherent way both administrative and medical information. The image of the hospital proposed by the system does not present any distortion (Figure 1) and both medical and administrative activity indicators have to be obtain as summarized statistics through relialable filters (Fetter's groups, drugs consumption rates, beds occupancy rates,...).

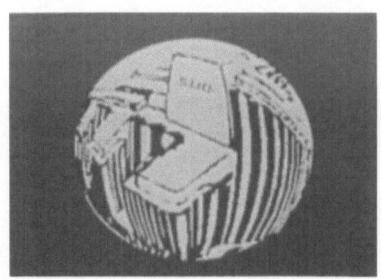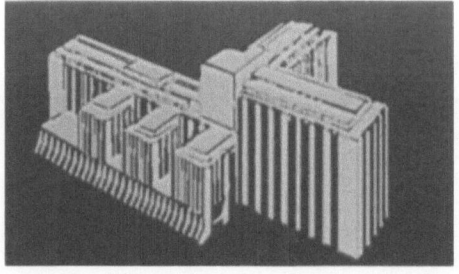

Figure 1 : distortion in the information sytem   coherence in the information system

Building such an IHIS needs different steps in its conception and specification life cycle :

A) the conception phase

1 - explicitation of the requirements of the future users

In this first step, we have used a method called RACINES [36], which gives a scheme leading interviews and meetings between future users and the conception team (Figure 2). Each human actor of the information system proposes his particular view, own needs and goals about the IHIS and the synthesis is validated on blackboards summarizing the creation, circulation, manipulation and storage of information and its principal treatments in the existing system. The systematic use of icons (symbolizing persons, buildings, information transmission roads, information treatment tools,...) allows in general an easy taking into account the description of the existing information system and permits the users feedback about the exact future requirements. In general, this approach corresponds to a top-down description of the information system : we have used at this step in Grenoble the DEC top-mapping method

"We have to improve the quality of the patient care"   "We need a better organization of the patient stay"

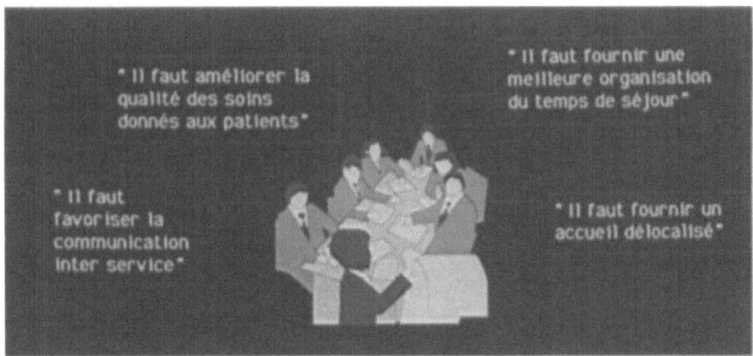

"We have to encourage the interservice communication"   "We want a delocalized patient reception"

Figure 2 :   needs and requirements expression meeting

2 - synoptic description of the data flows and processes

In this second step, we have used the SADT (or IDEF0) method : it consists in a top-mapping approach describing the processes (or actions) made on the data in a generative hierarchical frame from the general aspecific missions a hospital has to fulfil, to the very specific terminal actions made in a clinical or administrative service. If we take the department level (Figure 3), we can so successively list the various actions different units of a surgical department for example have to perform and we organize them in a logically dependent tasks sequence representing the SADT tree (Figure 4). In each box representing an action are mentioned input, output and control data, and also mechanisms used to process these data, the

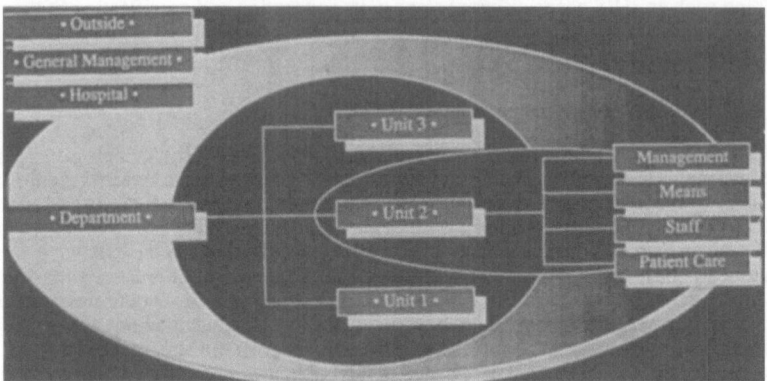

Figure 3 :   decomposition of the department level

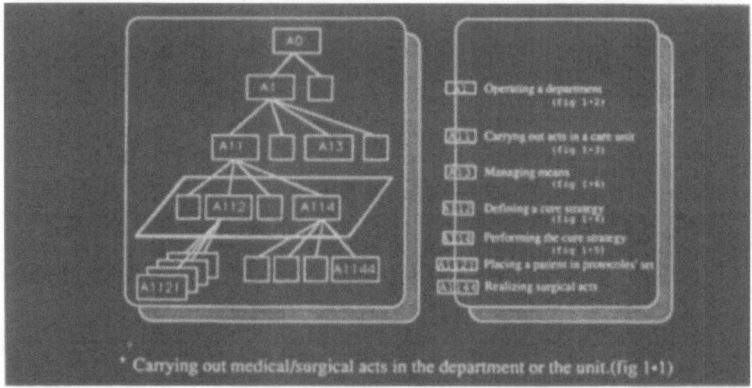

Figure 4 :   the SADT actions tree

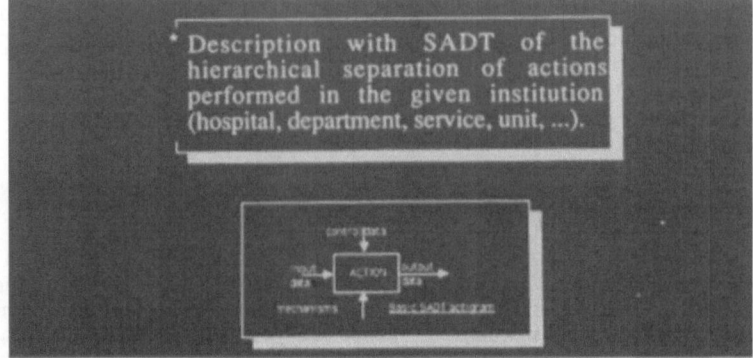

Figure 5 :   the SADT actigram

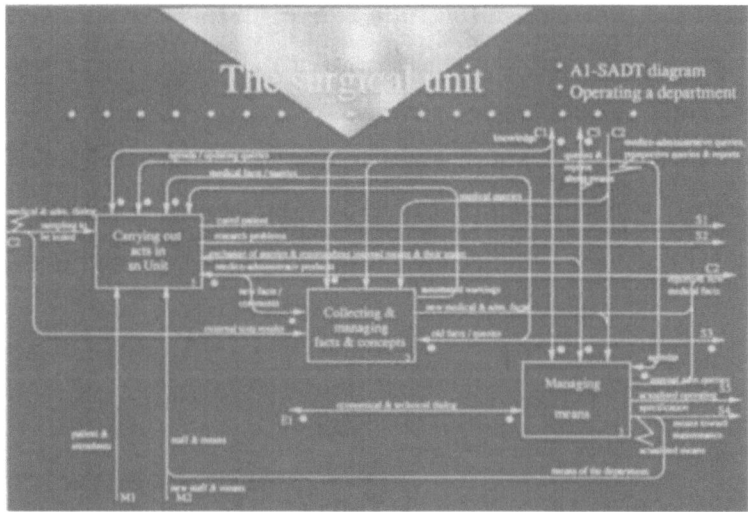

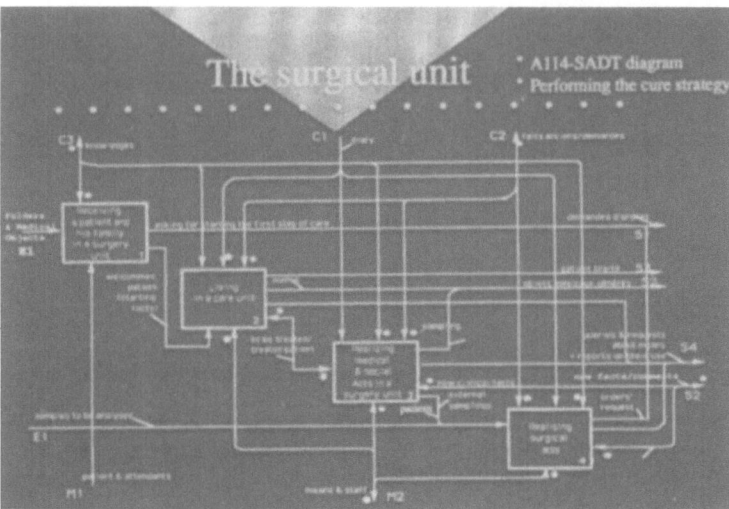

Figure 6 : description of the actigrams "Operating a department" (above) and "Performing a cure strategy" (below)

whole being called a SADT actigram (Figure 5). Each actigram can be precised as a collection of several subactigrams (see Figure 6 for the decomposition of the high level actigram "Operating a department" and of the preterminal actigram "Performing the cure strategy")

3 - synoptic description of the data flows and actors

In this third step, we have used a Yourdon-like method, which gives on the diagonal of a matrix the list of human actors involved in the hospital information system, and at the intersection of a row and a column the exchanged data between these actors (Figure 7). The description can be a top-down one, by considering at the beginning groups of actors (corresponding to the classical typology of the staff in a hospital) and after by considering a sub-matrix for such actors groups.

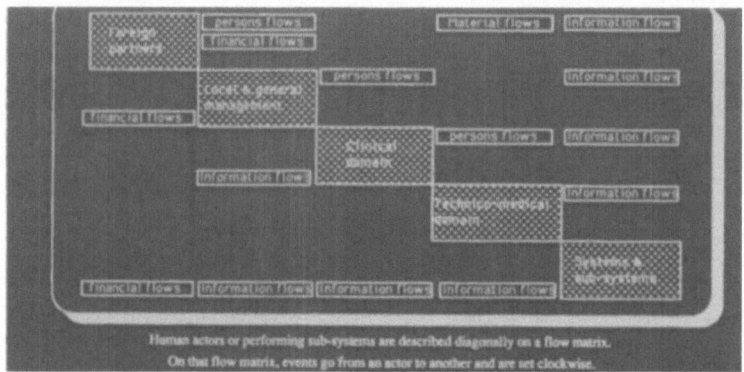

Figure 7 :   a Yourdon-like actor-data flow matrix

4 - functional description of workstations

In this fourth step, we have used a cross-approach between the two previous view, permitting an actor-centered description of the data processing. Figure 8 shows an example of such a functional description centered on surgeon outside and inside tasks [32,34]. For instance, we meet inside the operating theater different actors having close relations with the surgeon : patient, anaesthesist, assistant surgeon, instrumentalist nurse,... For example, the major actions processed under the responsability of the assistant surgeon are :

- perform preoperative measurements and observations
- manage the pre- and peroperative imaging (CAT-scanner, NMR, microscope, X-Ray, echography, laser acquisition,...)
- use an expert system to help certain therapeutic decisions
- ensure relationship with the preoperative or extemporaneous micropahologist.

Some specific functionalities permitted by technical improvements can appear at this stage, like the vocal command and control of surgical tools, or the peroperative display on specialized monitors of clinical information comming from the patient medical data files, or of encyclopedic information coming from surgical atlas or protocole books. The command and the control of a specific surgical robot can also represent such a new requirement to replace a systematic stereotactic procedure of making a biopsic puncture or setting a Curie-therapy needle in a precise location of the patient body.

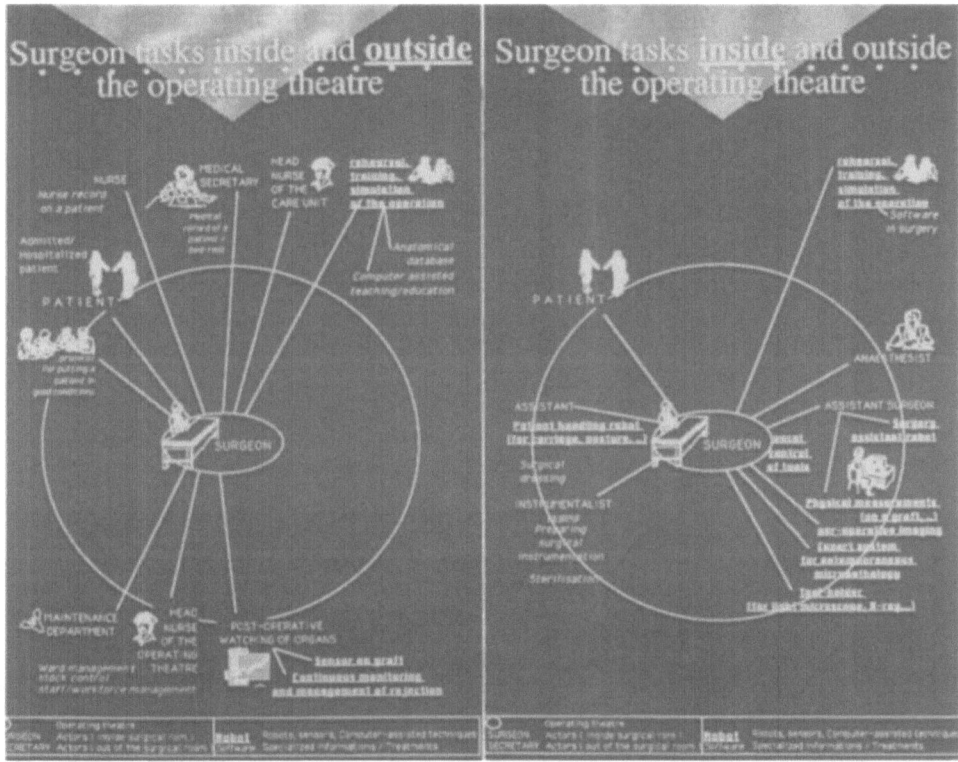

Figure 8 :   functional description of a surgeon workstation

B) the specification phase

1 - specification of applications on workstations

In this first step, we have used the Merise method. An example of required applications can be the specialized surgical record or the nursing care record (Figure 9), which need a precise specification before realizing a prototype in order to obtain the users feedback.

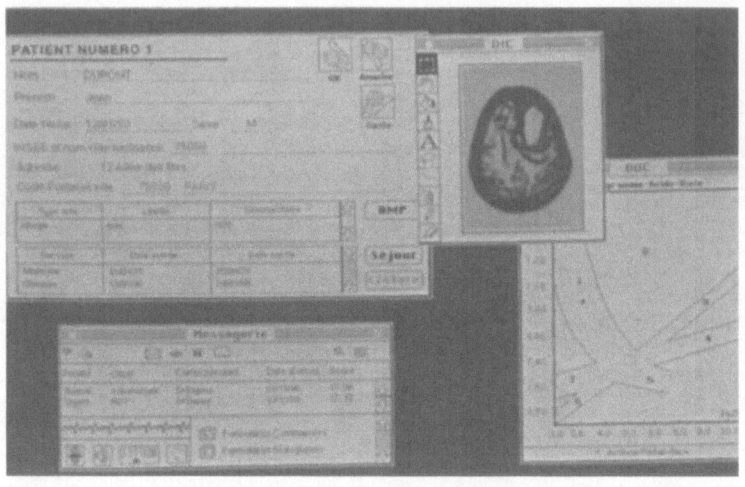

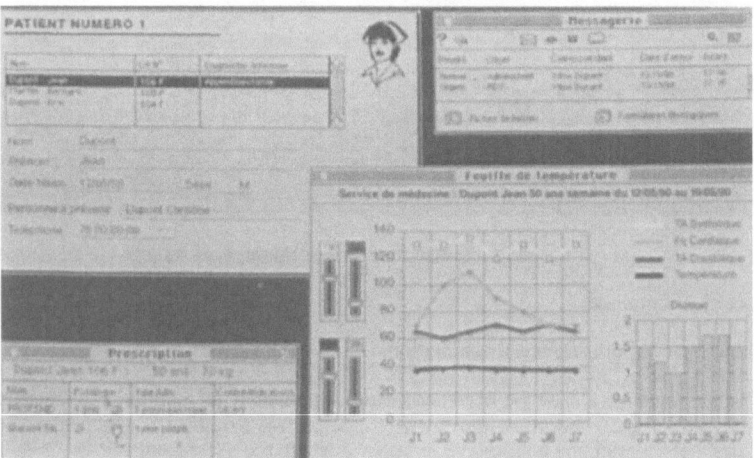

Figure 9 : Prototype screens for a specialized surgical record (above) and for a nursing care record (below)

2 - specification of globally constrained tasks

In this second step, we can use the Charme language [37] : it allows the taking into account of time constraints (leading to optimizing criteria like in linear programming) and can be useful in specification and prototyping applications like "agenda" management, "acta" storage, staff management, drug stocks dispatching,...

3 - specification of the integration tasks

In this third step, we are using the Merise method ; integration tasks require in particular :
- the building of interfaces between applications developed respectively on administrative (as the patient reception procedures) and on clinical (as the patient medical records) workstations
- the building of interfaces between communication protocols between different computer worlds (as in the DEC-IBMPC-Apple integration, by writing soft bridges between DecNet, TCPIP and AppleTalk)
- the building of interfaces between classical medical data bases (implemented in general in a DBMS) and the knowledge base of an expert system devoted to the medical decision making (implemented in a KBMS), in order for instance to estimate automatically the weights involved by an inference engine functioning in uncertain environment
- creation of common dictionaries of medico-administrative data and acts, common sets of formularies, and matching tools for a multimodality information coming from different sources (like medical anatomic and functional image devices, biological automata,...)
- creation of a minimum common living medical record following the patient during the same stay in the hospital between different services
- creation of a medico-administrative summarized record after the departure of the patient

4 - simulation of data creation, storage, exchange and manipulation

In this last step, we have used SADT simulation tools (we have also proposed the IDA-ISDOS method [28]) based on Petri nets approach. After quantifying the volumetry of data flows and timing of data processes, we can simulate the information exchanges and treatment in order to detect bottle-necks and critical limitant parameters of the information dynamics. These computer assisted simulation tools are especially necessary when no existing information system exists, and hence when we have no a priori calibration of the communication system.

2 Building a PACS

Medical images represent certainly in a hospital the most productive (in storage volume) source of information : for example, in the university hospital of Grenoble, the mean image volume of computerized images per patient is about 5 Mo. That corresponds to a global volume of 250 Go, for a total of about 50 000 patients pro year consulting services of numerical medical imaging (central radiology and neuroradiology with TDM, angiography, echography, and the NMR service). If we want have on line this information just for the 10 past years, we need a Mega-juke-box of about 1000 numerical optical disks. This volume will be multiplied by 5 when the numerical X-ray radiology will be generalized, involving a rapid hard access to the physical images and a fast logic querying to their corresponding logic images, i.e. the radiologic reports. In Grenoble, the design phase began in 1988 in the frame of the director scheme for informatizing of the university hospital. The actors were, after deciding to leave separate the public and the private (Multimed Race) Grenoble projects, the medical information department, all medical imaging services except paediatric radiology), the neurosurgery service, interested by the robotization of the stereotaxy and the radiotherapy service, interested by the problem of the inverse dosimetry and its automatization (cF. Figure 10 describing the present state of the Grenoble Image Information System GRENIS).

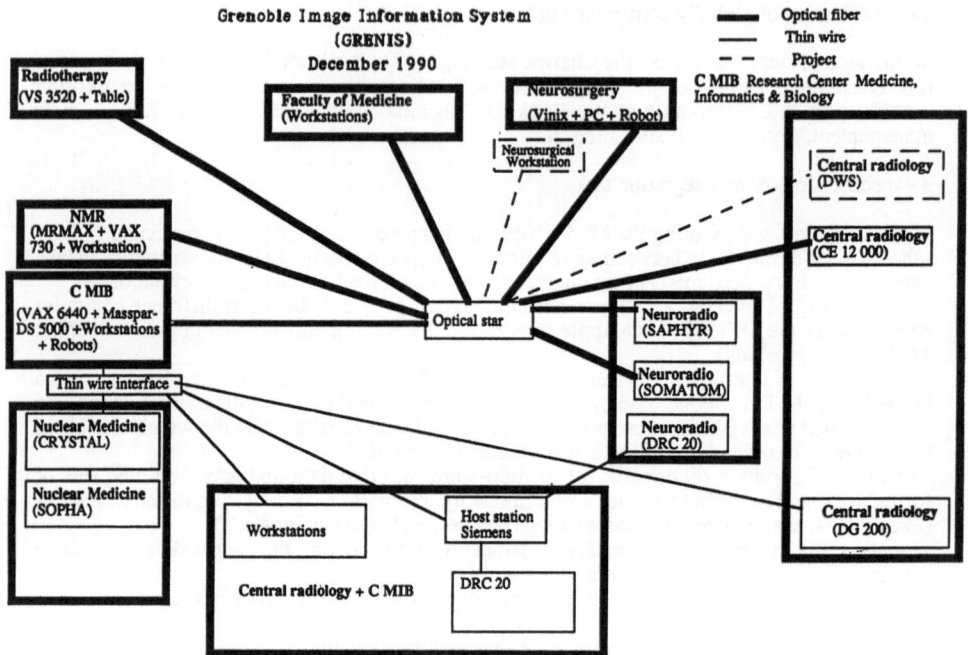

Figure 10 :   the present state ot the Grenoble Image Information System GRENIS

3 A surgeon oriented image workstation

An image information system integrating a Radiological Information System (RIS) [5] and other specific information systems devoted to nuclear medicine, functional neuro-imaging (magnetoencephalography, NMR spectrometry, pet-scan, fluorescent dye mapping,...) has to be interfaced with the general IHIS through dedicated workstations [6,7], which represent the concrete location of the integration. An example of such a workstation is a surgeon oriented image workstation.

Multimedia functions identified on this workstation are numerous : some already are supported by existing mechanisms (such as natural language interface, vocal interface, 3D reconstruction stereotactic robot, cf. for example [8,2,3,4,5,6,14]) and for others, mechanisms

of the computerized issue are to be found. Nevertheless, today's acquired knowledge makes it possible within the 5 next years.
These functions can be summed up as follows :
- consulting a medical folder enclosing multimedia images subfiles
- vocal and tactile command for tools
- intraoperative simulation of the action, by interactive 3D imaging
- consulting of multimedia databases enclosing operative protocols and anatomical atlas used as reference
- performing the surgical action and intra-operative decision making
- monitoring of the patient or of cut-off organs.

This conception approach allows to isolate and choose applications to be developed. One example is presented on Figure 11, on which we can see a fracture line impossible to detect on the TDM slices and shown by a 3D reconstruction. Another example is given on Figure 12, which shows a preoperative segmentation of the wrist (using a neural network enhancement technique) and the dynamical study of the 3D-reconstructed articulation. .

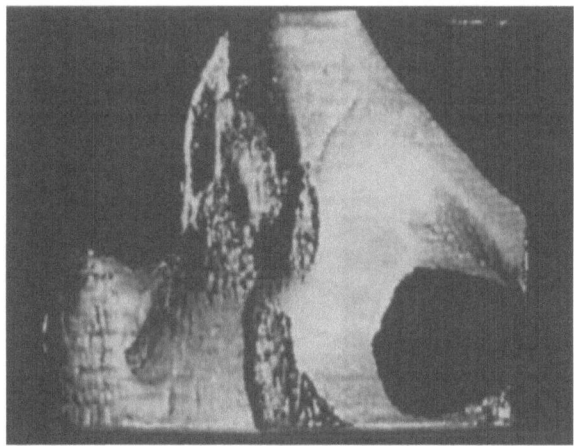

Figure 11 :   detection of a fracture line on a 3D reconstruction of the hip-bone

You will find hereafter some examples of on-going applications which may converge to the realization of a workstation able to help the surgical intervention, such as :
- automatized help to realize surgical interventions :
        . stereotactic neurosurgery [8-14], involving the 2D segmentation (Figure 13), the use of an atlas of the brain (Figure 14) and of a 6-axes robot designed by CAD (Figure 15) and able to make biopsic punctures (Figure 16) or deep electrodes or Curie-therapy needles setting (Figure 17)
        . computer-assisted intervertebral puncture [15,16]
        . pedicular screwing [17]
        . cranio-facial surgery [18] (Figure 18)
        . wrist surgery [19,20] (cf. Figure 12)
- matching of images from various origins, implying the knowledge of the peroperative referential (obtained through a laser acquisition for example as in Figure 19)
- definition of an atlas necessary to estimate relationships between normal (with areas to avoid) and pathological objects, and to use the localizing value of images in a diagnostic and therapeutic aim (Figure 14).

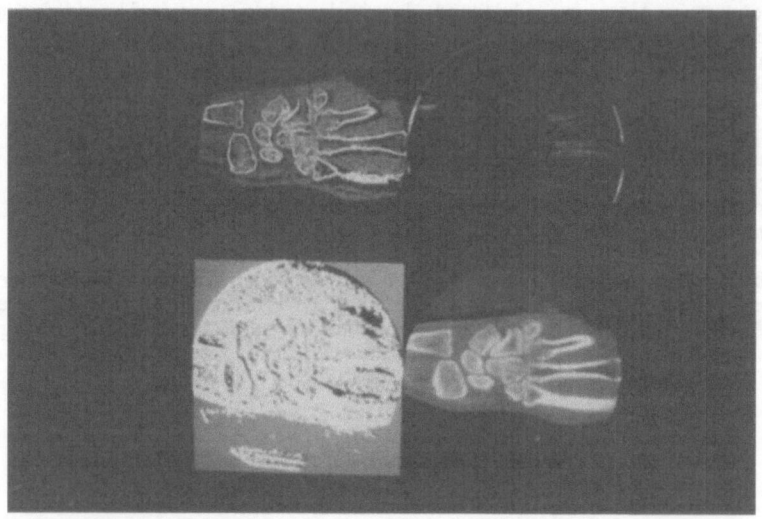

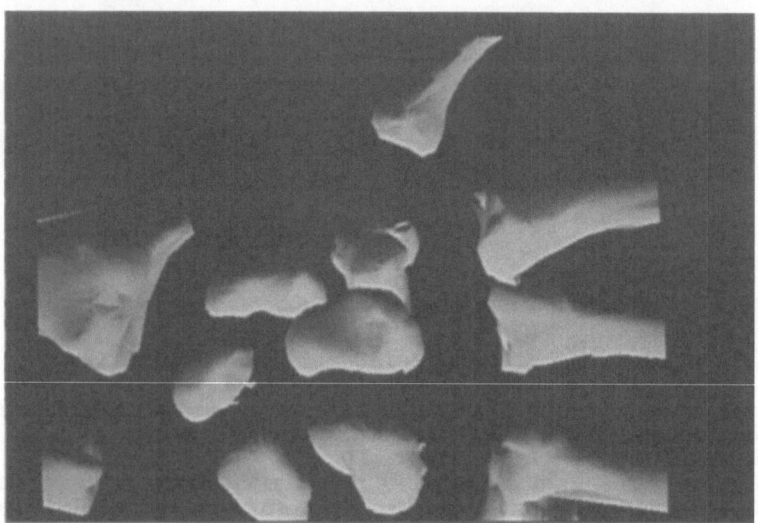

Figure 12 :   2D segmentation and 3D dynamical study of a wrist (from CAT-scanner slices)

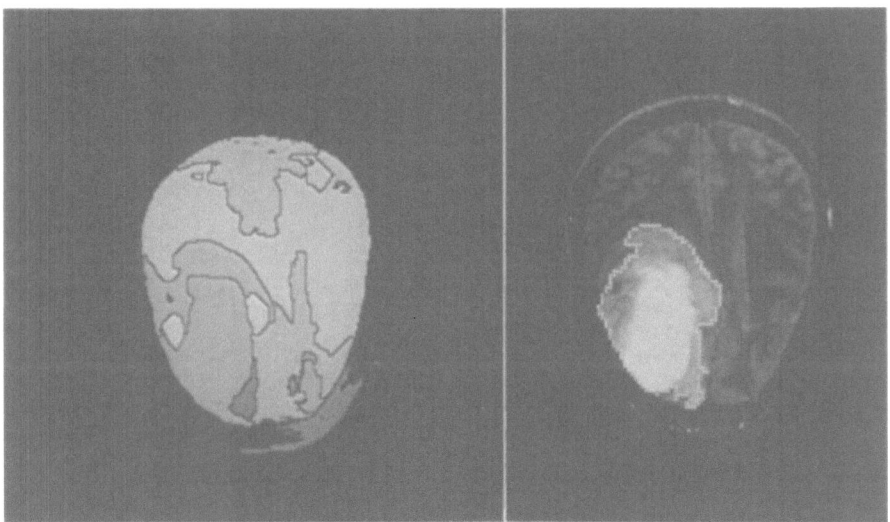

Figure 13 :   2D segmentation of a brain tumour (NMR image)

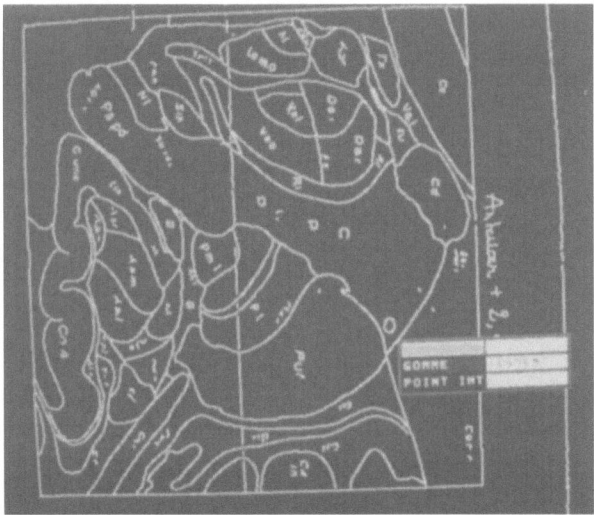

Figure 14 :   digitalization of a brain atlas

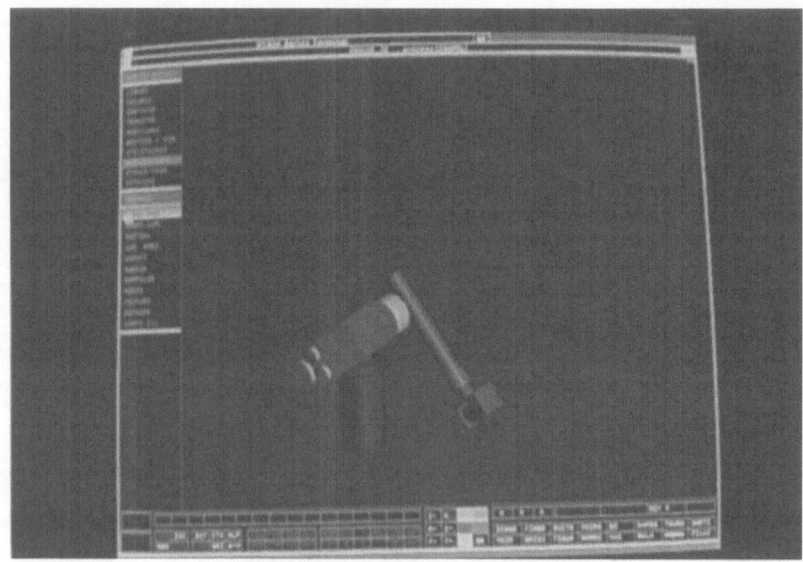

Figure 15 :   computer assisted design of a 6-axes robot

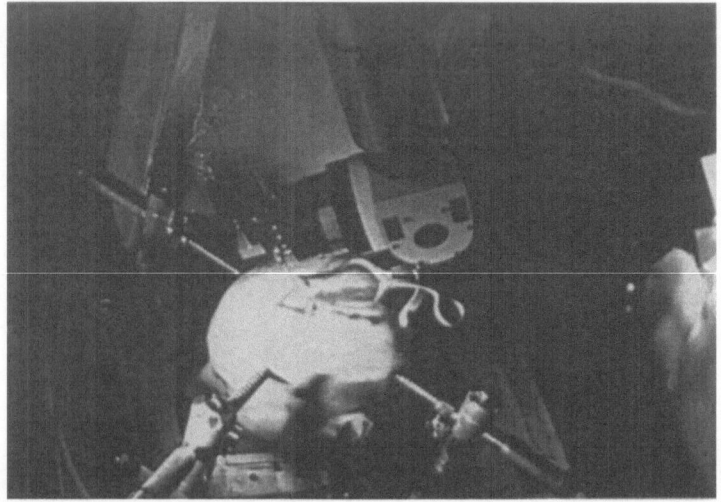

Figure 16 :   biopsic puncture made by the 6-axes robot

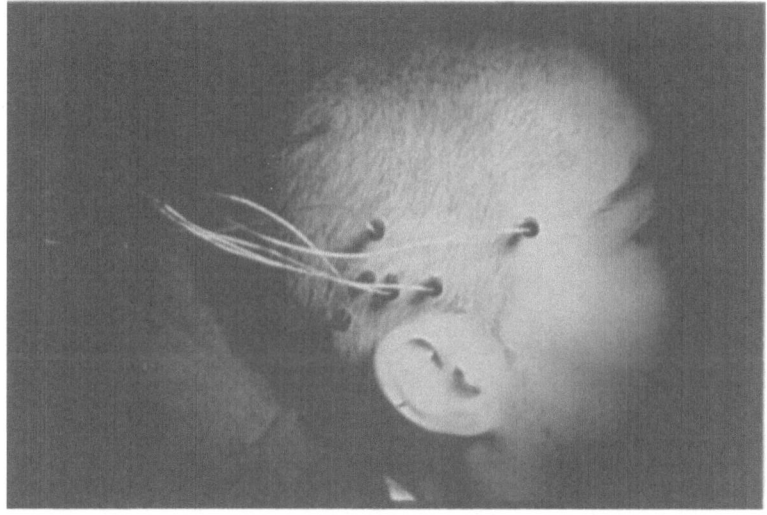

Figure 17 : deep electrodes setting by the robot for the Parkinson disease cure (Pr. A. Benabid)

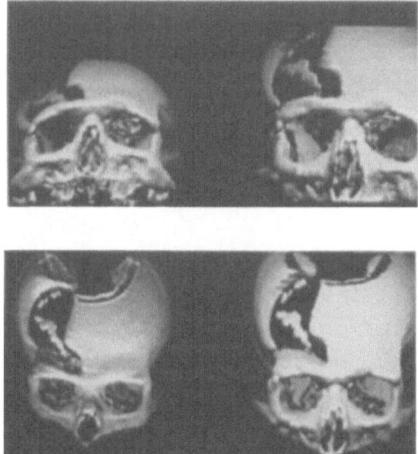

Figure 18 a :   pre-operative imaging for cranio-facial surgery

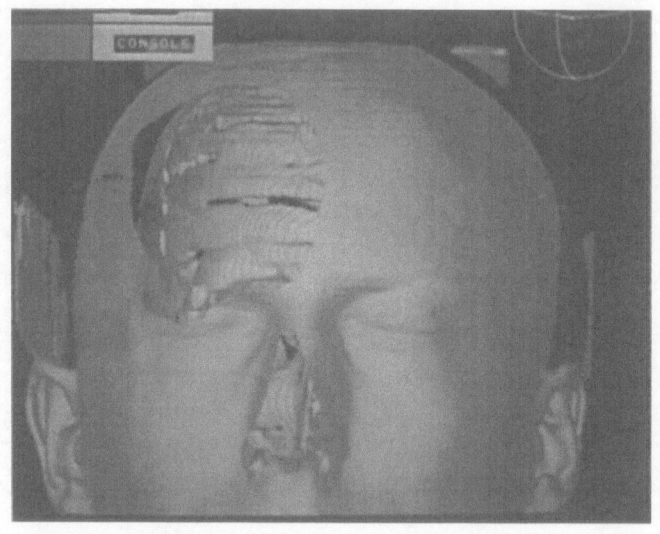

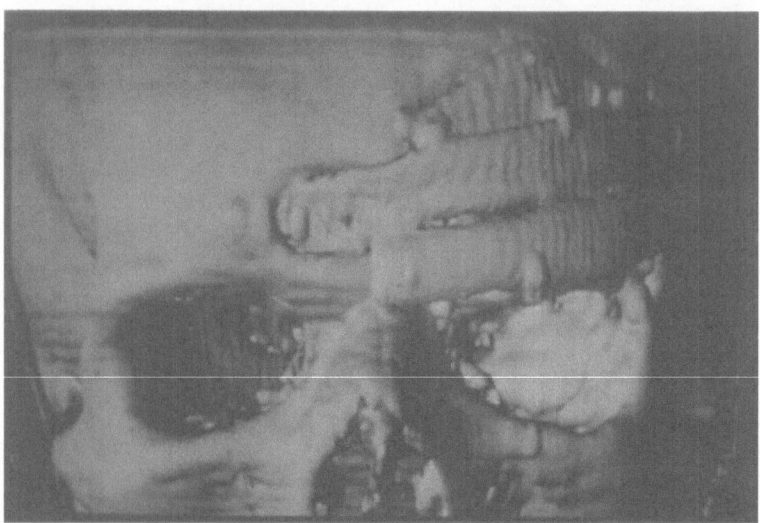

Figure 18 b :   post-operative imaging for cranio-facial surgery

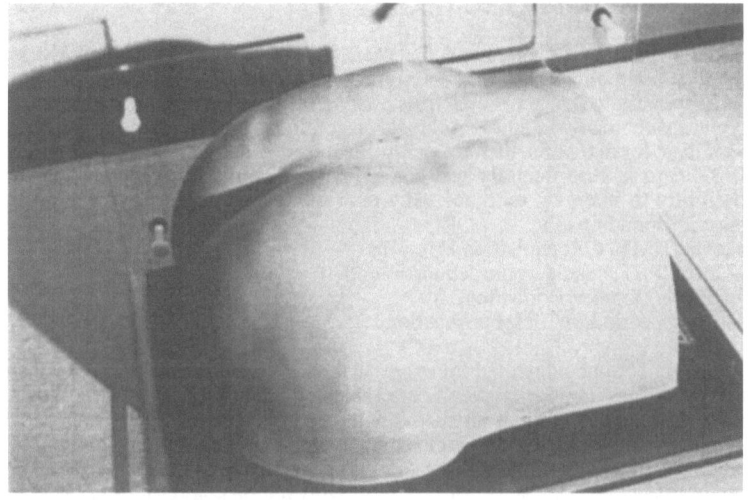

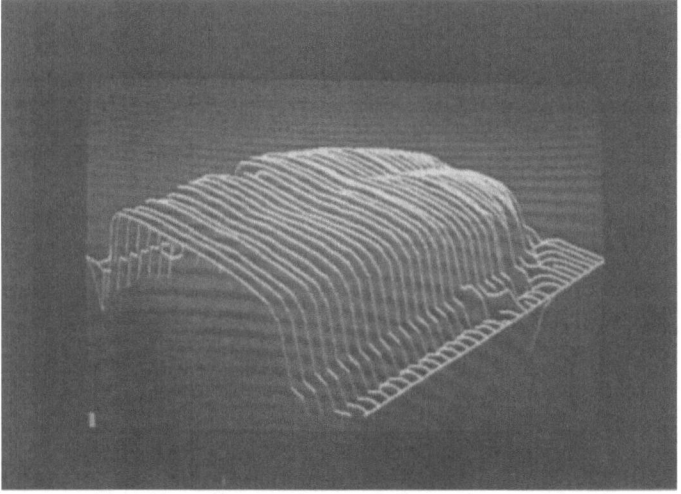

Figure 19 :   real-time laser acquisition of the back skin surface previous to a matching

4 Towards an ISCAMI

An Integrated System for Computer Aided Management and Manipulation of Medical Images has to permit the matching of multimodality images and clinical information. A clinician or a surgeon will be able to use multimodality images on this specific workstation in order to confront functional, anatomic and real time acquired images of the same organ together with other patient data, for diagnosis, therapy and medical education purposes. That implies :
1) the possibility to acquire precisely and rapidly images coming from different sources
2) the possibility to integrate with accuracy multimodality images by matching the patient referentials corresponding to :
anatomic level (NMR, CT acquisition,...)
functional level (PET, scintigraphic acquisition,...)
monitoring level (Doppler acquisition,...)
clinical and therapeutic level (laser acquisition,...)

This matching could be obtained for example through the correspondance of features (like geometric singularities, for example the crest or thalweg lines of the grey landscape as shown in Figure 20) of the medical object of interest. It will prepare the computer assistance to clinical or surgical therapies. Such an ISCAMI workstation could be able to acquire and treat in real time its own environment (Figure 21), in order to make possible the peroperative matching helping the guiding of medico-surgical acts. The ISCAMI workstation could for example constitute the key computer aided tool for a future computer assisted operating theater (Figure 22). It fulfils all general requirements of the surgeon workstation described above and is able to display for example on hanging monitors in the operating theater matched pre- and peroperative images, decisions proposed by expert systems, optimal trajectories extrapolated on the screen from the end of a surgical tool whose location has been acquired after laser scan,...

To conclude, an efficient ISCAMI workstation has to be connected through a PACS with all numerical image devices in a hospital : it will become the exact interface between the general IHIS and the final medical human actor (clinician or surgeon), allowing for a patient the synthesis of all past and present medical data (from the medico-administrative report to the real-time acquired and processed peroperative images).

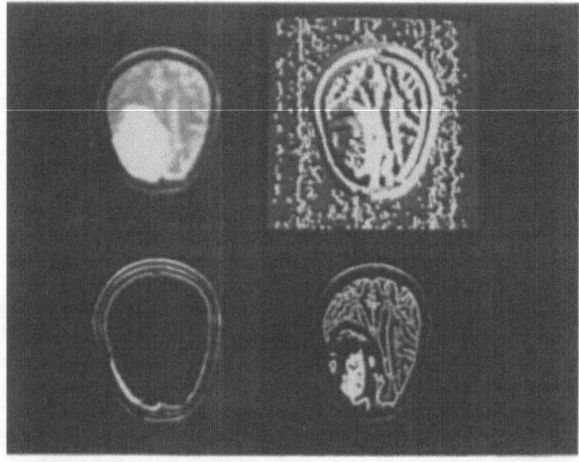

Figure 20   crest and thalweg lines of the grey landscape of a NMR image

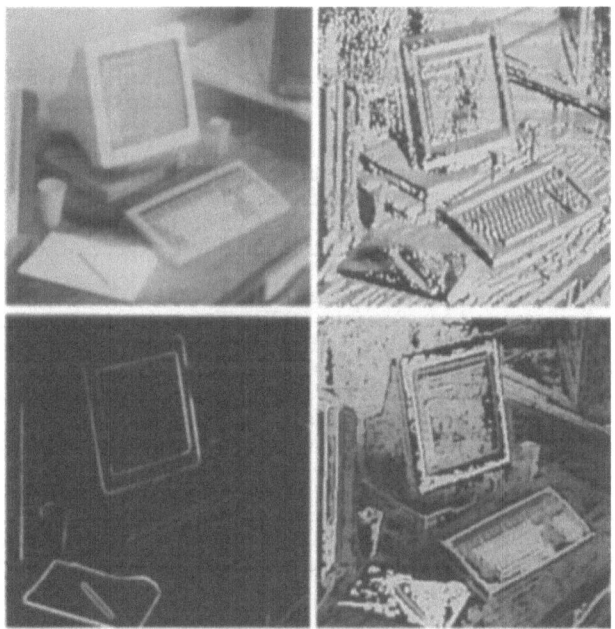

Figure 21 :   an ISCAMI workstation processing its own image

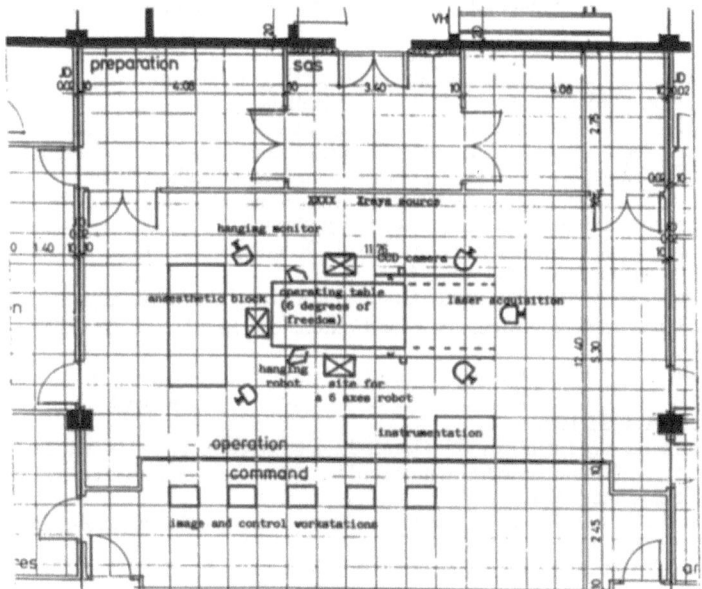

Figure 22 :   an example of a computer-assisted operating-theater

Acknowledgements

This work has been supported by an EERP research program of the DEC company.

References

[1]   Jost, R.G., W., Wessel, G.J., Blaine, J.R., Cox & R.L., Hill : PACS - Is there light at the end of the tunnel. In : Medical imaging III. PACS system design and evaluation. SPIE 1093, 74-84 (1989).

[2]   Lamarque, J.L., J.M., Bruel, H., Lestienne, P., Lopez & M., Gareil : PACS and medical selection imaging. In : Computer assisted radiology, Proceedings CAR 89, eds. H.U. Lemke, M.L. Rhodes, C.C. Jaffe & R. Felix, pp. 483. Berlin : Springer Verlag 1989.

[3]   Rienhoff, O. & K., Retter. PACS and HIS - A difficult marriage. In Computer assisted radiology, Proceedings CAR 89, eds. H.U. Lemke, M.L. Rhodes, C.C. Jaffe & R. Felix, pp. 493-495. Berlin : Springer Verlag 1987.

[4]   Gibaud, B., F., Picand, A., Benslimane, P., Grassin, L., Urbano, C., Toumoulin, F., Fresne, M., Rouvière & J.M., Scarabin : SIRENE : design and evaluation of a PACS prototype. In : Computer assisted radiology, Proceedings CAR 89, eds. H.U. Lemke, M.L. Rhodes, C.C. Jaffe & R. Felix, pp. 484-489. Berlin : Springer Verlag 1989.

[5]   Rienhoff, O. & C.F.C., Greinacher : A general PACS-RIS interface. Lecture Notes in Medical Informatics, Vol. 37. Berlin : Springer Verlag 1988.

[6]   Hunter, T.B. & K.M., McNeill : the radiologist workstation. Invest. Radiol. 25, 282-284 (1990).

[7]   Arenson, R.L., D.P., Chakraborty, S.B., Seshadri & H.L., Kundel : The digital imaging workstation. Radiology 176, 303-315 (1990).

[8]   Benabid, A., P., Cinquin, S., Lavallée, J.F., Le Bas, J., Demongeot, J., de Rougemont : A computer driven robot for stereotactic surgery connected to cat-scan magnetic resonance imaging. Technological design and preliminary results. J. Applied Neurophysiology 50, 153-154 (1987).

[9]   Marque, I., S., Lavallée, C., Goret-Lezy & P., Cinquin : Towards a 3-D medical image analysis system based on a continuous modelling. In : SCAR 90, eds.R.L. Arenson & R. M. Friedenberg, pp. 191-197. Carlsbad : Symposia Foundation 1990.

[10] Lavallée, S. & P., Cinquin : Computer assisted medical interventions. In : 3D-imaging in medicine, eds. K.H. Höhne, pp. 301-312. Berlin : Springer Verlag, Nato ASI Series F, Vol. 60 1990.

[11] Leitner F., I., Marque, F., Berthommier, T., Coll, O., Francois, P., Cinquin & J., Demongeot : Neural networks and image processing. In : From pixels to features II, ed. J.C. Simon, pp. 173-194 . Amsterdam : North Holland 1990.

[12] Lavallée, S., P., Cinquin, J., Demongeot, A.L., Benabid, I., Marque & M., Djaïd : Computer assisted interventionist imaging : the instance of stereotactic brain surgery. In : Medinfo 89, Singapore, pp. 613-617. Amsterdam : North Holland 1989.

[13] Lavallée, S., P., Cinquin, J., Demongeot, A.L., Benabid, I., Marque & M., Djaid : Computer assisted driving of a needle into the brain. In : Computer assisted radiology, Proceedings CAR 89, eds. H.U. Lemke, M.L. Rhodes, C.C. Jaffe & R. Felix, pp. 416-420. Berlin : Springer Verlag 1989.

[14] Lavallée, S. : A New System for Computer Assisted Brain Surgery. In : Proceedings 11th IEEE Engineering in Med. and Biol. Conference, Seattle, pp. 926-927. Piscataway : IEEE 1989.

[15] Lavallée, S., P., Cinquin, C., Goret, J., Demongeot, G., Crouzet & P., Peltié : Ponction assistée par ordinateur. In : Actes Congrès AFCET RFIA 87, Antibes, pp. 543-550. Paris : AFCET 1987.

[16] Cinquin, P., S., Lavallée, C., Goret, J., Demongeot, G., Crouzet & P., Peltié : Computer assisted intervertebral puncture. In : Proceedings MIE 87, eds. A. Serio et al., pp. 847-852. Rome : EFMI 1987.

[17] Mazier, B., S., Lavallée & P., Cinquin : Chirurgie de la colonne vertébrale assistée par ordinateur. ITBM 11, 55-62 (1990).

[18] Cinquin, P., J.C., Saget, G., Plasse & P., Antoine : Chirurgie plastique maxillofaciale assistée par ordinateur. In : Proceedings A. I. Biomed 86, pp. 95-99. Montpellier : CRIM 1986.

[19] Moutet, F., A., Chapel, P., Cinquin & L., Rose-Pitet : Imagerie du carpe en 3D. Ann. Radiol. 33, 128-133 (1990).

[20] Brunie, L. & S., Miguet : 3D reconstruction of the wrist : a new method of segmentation. DEA Report. Grenoble : IMAG 1989 and (submitted).

[21] Vermont, J., P., Cinquin & J., Demongeot : PACS and related research in France. In : PACS in Medicine, eds. B. Huang et al.. Amsterdam : North Holland, NATO ASI Series (to appear).

[22] Retter, K., A.J., Herbst & O., Rienhoff : Computer-assisted radiology : RIS/PACS. Attempts at definition and questions of interfacing (in this volume).

[23] Cinquin, P., J., Demongeot, M., Chabre-Peccoud & J.P., Giraudin : Analyse d'un système d'information hospitalier. In : Proceedings Euromédecine 86, pp. 135-142. Montpellier : Sauramps Médical 1986.

[24] Demongeot, J. & P., Cinquin : Perspectives de l'informatique médicale. In : Actes VIIIe Journées Francophones d'Informatique, pp. 79-100. Grenoble : IMAG 1986.

[25] Berrut, C., P., Cinquin, Y., Nie, G., Munoz, Y., Chiaramella, J., Demongeot & M., Coulomb : Modélisation sémantique de comptes rendus radiologiques. In : Actes du Congrès sur l'Intelligence Artificielle et Santé, pp. 191-200. Toulouse : SITEF 1987.

[26] Cinquin, P., C., Berrut, Y., Chiaramella, J., Demongeot & M., Coulomb : Interest of quasi-natural language reporting for medical images retrieving. In : Proceedings MIE 87, eds. A. Serio et al., pp. 872-877. Rome : EFMI 1987.

[27] Cinquin, P., J., Demongeot, M., Chabre-Peccoud & J.P., Giraudin : Specification of an integrated hospital information system with computer assisted information system design methods. In : Proceedings MIE 87, eds. A. Serio et al., pp. 31-35. Rome : EFMI 1987.

[28] Chabre-Peccoud, M., P., Cinquin & J., Demongeot : Modelling and simulation of an IHIS. In : Proceedings Working Conf. Towards new hospital information systems, ed. A. Bakker, pp. 245-252. Amsterdam : North Holland 1988.

[29] Berthommier, F., J., Demongeot & J.L., Schwartz : A neural net for processing of stationary signals in the auditory system. In : IEE Proc. Conf. Signal Proc. London , pp. 287-291. London : IEE 1989.

[30] Hervé, T., J.M., Dolmazon & J., Demongeot : Random field and neural information : a new representation for multi-neuronal activity. Proc. Natl. Acad. Sc. 87, 806-810 (1990).

[31] Cinquin, P., S., Lavallee & J., Demongeot : A new system for computer assisted neurosurgery. In : IARP Medical and Helthcare Robotics Newcastle, pp. 63-66. London : DTI 1989.

[32] Weil, G., J., Vermont, F., Moutet & J., Demongeot : Conception d'un poste de travail chirurgical informatisé. In : Informatique et Imagerie Médicale. Journées Francophones d'Informatique Médicale de Nîmes, pp. 53-63. Rennes : ENSP 1990.

[33] Berthommier, F., O., Francois, D., Francillard, T., Coll, P., Cinquin, I., Marque & J., Demongeot : Asymptotic behavior of neural networks and image processing. In : Self-Organization, Emerging properties and Learning, ed. A. Babloyantz. New York : Plenum Press, NATO Series to appear.

[34] Vermont, J., P., Cinquin & J., Demongeot : PACS and related research in France. In : PACS in Medicine, eds. B. Huang et al. Amsterdam : North Holland, NATO ASI Series to appear.

[35] Cinquin, P. & J., Demongeot : Medical imaging evaluation in ISCAMI. In : NATO Conf. on medical evaluation Montpellier, ed. F. Grémy. New York : Plenum Press to appear.

[36] Racines, ed. MRI Mission à l'Informatique, tome I & II. Paris : La Documentation Française 1982.

[37] Weil, G. : L'hôpital au service du malade. Transfert des concepts, des méthodes, des outils de la gestion de production. In : Informatique et Imagerie Médicale. Journées Francophones d'Informatique Médicale de Nîmes, pp. 447-454. Rennes : ENSP 1990.

[38] Cinquin, P. & S., Lavallée : Gestes médicaux et chirurgicaux assistés par ordinateur : bases méthodologiques. In : Informatique et Imagerie Médicale. Journées Francophones d'Informatique Médicale de Nîmes, pp. 65-75. Rennes : ENSP 1990.

Index of Authors

Achevé d'imprimer par ⬛ Corlet, Imprimeur, S.A.
14110 Condé-sur-Noireau (France)
N° d'Éditeur : 297 - N° d'Imprimeur : 1529/BF - Dépôt légal : juillet 1991

Imprimé en C.E.E.